The Teen's Coping Toolkit

Navigate Social Pressures, Manage Difficult Situations, and Build Self-Esteem

C.M. Krueger, PhD

Contents

Introduction

Have you ever felt like your emotions are a rollercoaster—up one minute and plummeting the next? Or perhaps there are days when it feels like stress and anxiety are your constant companions, making even the simplest tasks seem overwhelming. You're not alone. Let's face it; today's teens face a unique set of emotional challenges, and the need for effective coping strategies has never been more urgent. Recent studies show a significant rise in mental health issues among teenagers, which shines an even brighter light on the importance of accessible and practical tools for managing emotions.

The Teen's Coping Toolkit: Navigate Social Pressures, Manage Difficult Situations, and Build Self-Esteem is designed to offer practical strategies that you can use to handle the twists and turns of the never-ending rollercoaster that is your teenage years. This book isn't just for flipping through; it's a tool to make psychology work for you, breaking down complex theories into bite-sized, applicable steps that fit right into your daily routine.

While I primarily wrote this book with you, the teenager, in mind, it's also a valuable resource for the adults in your life. Whether they're parents, teachers, or counselors, the extra bit of insight into what you're going through and how they can support you can make all the difference in their general understanding. This two-sided perspective will enrich the conversation around emotional well-being, bridging the gap between generations and fostering mutual understanding.

This book is rooted in several therapeutic approaches, providing insights from methods including Cognitive Behavioral Therapy (CBT) and Dialectical Behavioral Therapy (DBT). These frameworks provide a foundation for the practical exercises sprinkled throughout the chapters —exercises that are simple, quick, and designed to be seam-lessly integrated into your everyday life. Each chapter addresses different emotions and scenarios you might encounter, from dealing with anxiety and stress to managing anger and battling depression—and the practical tools to meet you in the approach.

As you work through these pages, expect to be captivated by a compassionate and inspiring tone. This is not simply a manual; rather, think of it as a conversation with a friend who "gets it"—all the struggles, frustrations, and triumphs of teenage life. My goal is to empower you with self-regulation tools that help you manage your emotional world, take charge of your well-being, and succeed on your terms.

So, let's explore these pages together. Remember that this book is about your journey, challenges, and victories, but more than this, it's about equipping you with the knowledge and skills to face life's challenges with confidence and resilience. So, what are we waiting for? Let's start this journey together, turning the page toward a more empowered and emotionally intelligent you.

Chapter 1
Understanding Your Emotional Landscape

Have you ever stopped in your tracks because a sudden rush of anxiety left you breathless or felt your stomach tie itself into knots before a big presentation? These moments aren't just random; they're signposts, or in more simple terms—they are acting as your body's way of signaling your current emotional state.

Emotions aren't simply feelings; they are complex reactions that involve your body, mind, and environment, influencing and being influenced by each. This chapter will guide you through understanding these reactions, helping you recognize and interpret what your body and mind are trying to tell you through emotional signals. By becoming fluent in the language of your emotions, you'll be equipped to navigate the complexities of your daily life with greater ease and insight.

1.1 Decoding Emotional Signals: What Your Feelings Are Trying to Tell You

Our emotions can sometimes feel like mysterious forces taking over our bodies and minds, leaving us feeling helpless and out of control. But emotions aren't random—they're insightful messages that can reveal our deepest needs, desires, and values if we learn to decode them. Let's dive into how to interpret these messages, starting with the physical signs.

Identify Physical Signs of Emotions

Every emotion manifests physically in some way—whether it's the tension in your shoulders when you're anxious, the rapid heartbeat of excitement, or the heavy feeling in your limbs when you're sad. These sensations are your body's initial reactions to your emotional state, acting as the first indicators that something significant is happening internally. For instance, anxiety might make your stomach churn, and anger might make your hands clench or your jaw tighten. Recognizing these physical signs is crucial because they are the first clue to your internal feelings before you can even put a name to them. By paying attention to these physical cues, you can catch emotions early and address them before they become too overwhelming.

Link Emotions to Thoughts and Events

Once you notice these physical signs, the next step is to connect them to what's happening in your life. Emotions don't just pop up out of nowhere—they're usually sparked by thoughts or events. For example, that knot in your stomach before a test? It's probably tied to worries about how you'll perform or what the outcome might be. Or the sudden tension in your shoulders during a family dinner might be because you're stressed about potential conflicts or just want everyone to get along.

By figuring out what thoughts or events trigger your emotional reactions, you can start to predict and manage your responses better. This helps you keep your emotions in check and empowers you to handle the situations that cause them.

Understanding Emotional Reactions as Messages

All emotional responses you experience are packed with information about your values, boundaries, and needs. Anger, for instance, often signals that a boundary has been crossed or an individual value has been violated. Similarly, sadness can indicate a loss or a disconnect from something important to you.

By interpreting these emotions as messages rather than random outbursts, you can uncover what truly matters to you and guide your decisions and actions. This realization can transform how you view your emotional world, turning emotions from confusing reactions into meaningful insights that can help you navigate your life.

Practice Interpreting These Signals

To get better at figuring out what your emotions are telling you, make reflection a daily habit. Spend a few minutes each day thinking about any strong emotions you felt. Jot down the physical sensations you noticed, the snapshot of the situation you were in, and the thoughts running through your mind. This practice helps you connect the dots between your feelings, thoughts, and what's happening around you. The more you do this, the better you'll get at recognizing and managing your emotions, making sure they help rather than hinder your day.

Emotional Journaling Exercise

Try keeping an emotional journal to track your feelings in a structured way. Each day, write down significant emotional moments, focusing on what you felt physically, your thoughts, and what was happening around you.

This can be super insightful, helping you spot patterns in your emotional responses and triggers. Over time, your journal will become a handy tool in your emotional toolkit, offering clear insights to guide your personal growth and emotional management.

Remember, navigating your emotional landscape isn't about ignoring your feelings but understanding and managing them as crucial parts of your human experience. By getting good at interpreting what your emotions are saying, you'll empower yourself to lead a more balanced and fulfilling life.

1.2 The Science of Emotions: Understanding How and Why We Feel

Emotions are those quick responses we have to everything going on around us, and they're deeply tied to how our brain works. Understanding emotions starts with looking at the brain, especially the limbic system. This part of your brain isn't working solo—it's like the HQ for emotional processing. The limbic system has key players like the amygdala, hippocampus, and hypothalamus, which are super important in handling our emotional reactions.

Structures

The leading players in your emotional brain are:

The Amygdala: This almond-shaped structure is your emotional smoke alarm. It's specially tuned to detect potential threats and trigger your fight-or-flight response.

The Hippocampus: Think of this as your brain's librarian. It helps store and retrieve memories, which play a big role in how you react emotionally to situations.

The Prefrontal Cortex: This is the wise elder of your brain. It helps regulate your emotions and make rational decisions. It's still developing in teens, which explains a lot.

Meanwhile, chemicals called neurotransmitters and hormones start flooding your system. It's like your body's throwing a chemical rave, and your emotions are the unexpected guests. Some key players are:

Dopamine: The "feel-good" chemical that makes you feel rewarded and motivated.

Serotonin: Often called the "happiness hormone," it helps regulate mood.

Cortisol: The stress hormone that gets you ready for action in tough situations.

Oxytocin: The "love hormone" that helps with bonding and trust.

Chemical Aspects

Moving beyond the structures, let's delve into the chemical aspect of how we feel. Neurotransmitters, the brain's chemical messengers, profoundly impact our moods and emotions. Serotonin and dopamine are particularly influential. Serotonin helps regulate mood, appetite, and sleep, all of which influence our well-being.

Low levels of serotonin are linked with feelings of depression and anxiety. Dopamine, often called the 'feel-good' neurotransmitter, plays a significant role in how we experience pleasure and satisfaction. It's critical to our reward pathways, which are crucial for motivation and behaviors driven by pleasure. These neurotransmitters don't work alone. They interact within a huge, dynamic network, influencing and being influenced by other biochemical processes in our bodies.

Evolution and Survival

The evolutionary perspective on emotions reveals their fundamental role in survival. Consider the emotion of fear leading to a fight-or-flight response. This reaction is an evolutionary development designed to enhance our survival when we face threatening situations. When faced with danger, our bodies become flooded with hormones like adrenaline and cortisol, which work to prepare us to either fight the threat or flee to safety. The fight-or-flight response was crucial in prehistoric times when physical threats were common. Today, this same response kicks in during modern situations, like speaking in front of a crowd or during a tense moment in a game. Understanding this reaction helps us see that these intense emotions aren't just overreactions. They are deeply embedded responses that have helped humans survive for thousands of years.

Did you know that our emotional responses are also significantly influenced by the environment that surrounds us? Everything from the lighting in a room to the noise level in a cafe can affect how we feel. For instance, bright, harsh lighting can increase feelings of anxiety and stress, while soft, warm lighting can make us feel calm and relaxed.

Sounds play a similar role. The constant hum of city traffic can be stressful, while the sounds of nature can be soothing. Social settings also profoundly impact our emotions. Being surrounded by supportive friends can uplift our spirits, while feeling isolated or facing conflict in social interactions might trigger feelings of stress and sadness. Understanding these environmental impacts can help us make conscious choices about our surroundings to support our emotional well-being.

Navigating the complexities of our emotional brain might seem daunting, but understanding the basics of how emotions function biologically and chemically, their evolutionary purposes, and how external factors influence them provides a robust framework for us to do so.

With this knowledge, you can better manage your emotional responses as they relate to various situations, which can help you make informed decisions about interacting with the world around you as you maintain emotional balance and enhance your quality of life.

The Body-Emotion Connection

Here's a cool trick: your body can give you clues about what you're feeling. It's like your emotions are playing charades with your physical sensations:

- Butterfly stomach? You might be nervous or excited.
- Clenched fists? Anger might be knocking at your door.
- Heavy limbs? Sadness could be weighing you down.
- Racing heart? Hello, anxiety (or maybe you just ran up the stairs).
- Warm, tingly feeling? Could be happiness or love.

- Tense shoulders? Stress might be paying a visit.

1.3 Emotion or Mood: Recognizing the Difference

Understanding the distinction between your emotions and your moods is like learning the difference between weather and climate. Emotions are a lot like the weather: Intense and responsive to immediate surroundings, changing rapidly with conditions—sunshine brightening your day, or a storm cloud darkening your mood momentarily.

On the other hand, your moods are akin to climate: They are more enduring, less tied to specific events, and can influence your environment over a more extended period of time. Understanding this difference helps to identify what you are experiencing at any moment and equips you with strategies to manage these feelings effectively.

Define Emotions and Moods

Emotions are immediate, intense reactions to external stimuli. For instance, receiving praise from a teacher may spark joy, while harsh words from a peer might ignite anger. These reactions are typically brief, lasting from a few seconds to several hours, and are directly linked to a specific moment in time. Moods, on the other hand, are more sustained emotional states that do not necessarily have a direct trigger.

They can last for days or even weeks, coloring all experiences during that time. For example, you might feel a general melancholy for several days without an apparent reason, which may, in turn, affect how you perceive interactions and events around you.

Identifying the Duration and Triggers

To figure out if you're dealing with an emotion or a mood, look at how long it lasts and what triggered it. Emotions pop up quickly and are usually tied to a specific event, like feeling anxious before a test. Moods, on the other hand, last longer and aren't always linked to one clear cause. If you're feeling down and can't really pinpoint why, you're probably in a mood.

Recognizing these patterns is crucial in managing them effectively, as the strategies for dealing with fleeting emotions differ from those used to alter a prolonged mood.

Impacts on Thought and Behavior

Both emotions and moods significantly influence your thoughts and actions but require different approaches for management. Intense emotions can lead to impulsive decisions or reactions, like snapping at a friend in anger.

In contrast, a mood might subtly skew your perspective over time, potentially leading to prolonged feelings of pessimism or overly optimistic expectations. Managing emotions often requires immediate techniques to calm down and gain perspective, such as deep breathing or taking a moment to assess the reality of the situation. Moods typically need more sustained strategies, like engaging in regular exercise, seeking social interaction, or practicing mindfulness to shift your overall emotional baseline.

Emotional Triggers: What Sets You Off?

Emotional triggers are like the "on" switch for different emotions. Some common triggers include:

- Stress
- Conflicts with friends or family
- Changes in your routine
- Lack of sleep
- Certain places or situations
- Social media
- Memories of past events
- Criticism or praise from others

Everyone's triggers are different. What stresses you out might be no big deal for your friend, and vice versa. The key is to start noticing your own personal triggers.

Real-life Application

Consider a typical week in your life where you encounter various situations at school, at home, or during leisure activities. Let's say you felt a sudden surge of happiness when you scored well on a test—that's an emotion. Later in the week, you might notice a lingering feeling of sadness without an apparent reason, affecting your motivation and interaction with friends—that's a mood.

Try keeping a simple log for a week to take note and practice categorizing your feelings. Jot down brief descriptions of significant emotional reactions, as well as your ongoing feelings each day. Review your notes at the end of each week to identify which entries describe emotions that are linked to specific events and which represent moods without a direct cause. This practice will enhance your overall awareness and general understanding of your emotional patterns, which may enable you to apply appropriate coping strategies effectively.

By learning to both differentiate and appropriately respond to emotions and moods, you will gain crucial skills in emotional self-regulation. These skills help in personal growth and achieving emotional balance and can empower you to navigate the complexities of relationships and daily challenges more effectively.

With practice, you'll begin to manage life's ups and downs with greater ease and flexibility, leading to a healthier, more fulfilling life experience.

1.4 Developing an Emotional Vocabulary: Beyond Happy and Sad

Expanding your emotional vocabulary is like adding more colors to your palette in art class. It gives you a more prosperous, more nuanced way to express and understand your feelings. Many limit themselves to basic terms like "happy" or "sad," but emotions are far more complex than that.

Think about the difference between feeling "frustrated" versus "enraged" or "content" versus "elated." Each word paints a specific picture of your emotional state and can guide you in understanding and responding to your feelings more effectively.

Expand Emotional Language

Let's introduce a broader range of "emotion" words to expand your emotional vocabulary. Are you feeling content, pleased, joyful, or thrilled when you feel happy? Keep in mind that each word has a slightly different connotation and intensity. Similarly, sadness can range from feeling blue or melancholy to feeling sad or grief-stricken.

By naming your emotions more precisely, you begin to gain clarity about your thoughts, which is the first step in managing your emotions effectively. This precision helps in self-understanding and improves communication with others, as it allows you to convey your emotional state more accurately, reducing misunderstandings and fostering better relationships.

Contextualizing Emotions

Understanding the context is key because it can change how you perceive an emotion. For example, the physical feelings of excitement and anxiety are pretty similar—both can make your heart race, palms sweat, and adrenaline surge, but the context makes all the difference—excitement before going on stage for a play versus anxiety before a big exam.

Knowing how context affects your emotions can help you reframe how you feel and react better. It's about asking yourself, "Why do I feel this way right now?" and thinking about what's happening around you that might be influencing your emotions.

The Feelings Wheel is a practical tool to help you expand and contextualize your emotional vocabulary. This visual aid displays many emotions stemming from core feelings like sadness, anger, fear, enjoyment, love, and surprise. Each core emotion branches into more specific feelings, helping you pinpoint exactly what you are experiencing. For instance, if you start with 'anger' on the wheel, you dive a little deeper to notice what you are actually feeling might feel 'irritated,' 'disgusted,' or 'furious.'

Using a Feelings Wheel not only aids in identifying and labeling your emotions, but also in understanding how they relate to one another and the root of your feelings.

Practice Through Daily Logs

Maintaining a daily emotional log can greatly enhance mastery of this expanded emotional vocabulary. Each day, take a few minutes to reflect on your emotional experiences and write them down. Describe the scenarios and label your emotions using specific words from your enhanced vocabulary.

Did a conversation with a friend leave you feeling rejuvenated, or did a comment from someone make you feel invalidated? Writing these details can help you see patterns over time, providing insights into how your emotions interact with and respond to your daily activities and relationships. This practice boosts your emotional intelligence and serves as a valuable self-reflection tool, helping you navigate your emotional world with greater awareness and precision.

You can change how you handle emotions by trying a few things: Expanding your emotional vocabulary, understanding how context affects your feelings, using tools like the Feelings Wheel, and keeping an emotional log. Having a richer emotional vocabulary helps you connect better with yourself and others, creating a more empathetic and understanding environment. As you get better at recognizing and talking about your feelings, you'll find it easier to navigate life's ups and downs.

1.5 Mapping Your Emotional Triggers and Responses

Understanding what triggers your emotions and how you react to these triggers is like having a roadmap for navigating your emotional landscape. Just as a driver might use GPS to avoid roadblocks and find the best route, you can use knowledge of your emotional triggers to manage your reactions and maintain control over your feelings. This understanding is crucial, as it helps you anticipate and prepare for emotional responses, allowing you to handle them more effectively when they arise.

The Emotional Intensity Scale

Emotions aren't just "on" or "off." They come in different intensities, like a volume knob for your feelings.

Try rating your emotions on a scale from one to ten:

1 = Barely noticeable (like a whisper)

5 = Definitely there, but manageable (normal speaking voice)

10 = Off the charts intense (rock concert level)

This can help you track how your emotions change over time and figure out when you might need to use some coping strategies.

Identify Triggers

The first step in mapping your emotional responses is identifying what triggers them. Triggers are specific situations, people, or thoughts that spark a particular emotional response in you.

For many teens, common triggers include:

- Stressful academic environments
- Conflicts with friends or family members
- Significant life changes, like moving to a new school or dealing with parents' divorce

For example, you might notice that you feel unusually irritable after spending long hours on schoolwork without breaks, or you might feel anxious when you think about speaking in front of your classmates. By pinpointing these triggers, you can begin to understand why you react in specific ways and start to address the underlying causes of your emotional responses.

Patterns of Emotional Response

Once you've identified your triggers, the next step is to observe how you typically respond to them. Do you withdraw and isolate yourself when you feel overwhelmed or react outwardly with anger or frustration? Tracking your responses over time can help you see patterns in your behavior. Whenever you interact with a friend who tends to be critical, you feel down for the rest of the day.

Recognizing these patterns is crucial because it allows you to predict and prepare for your reactions, allowing you to potentially pause and choose a different response in the future.

Developing Personal Strategies

Knowing your triggers and understanding your typical emotional responses is a game changer. It allows you to develop strategies for managing your reactions. Here are some simple but effective techniques you can try:

Take Deep Breaths: When you feel yourself getting overwhelmed, try taking a few deep breaths. This can help calm your nervous system and give you a moment to collect your thoughts.

Step Away from Stress: If you're in a stressful situation, sometimes the best thing to do is step away for a bit. Whether it's going for a short walk, finding a quiet spot, or just taking a break, this can help you gain some perspective.

Talk to Someone You Trust: Sharing your feelings with a friend, family member, or therapist can be incredibly helpful. They can offer support, advice, or just a listening ear, which can make a big difference.

Use a Feelings Wheel: A Feelings Wheel can help you pinpoint exactly what you're feeling, which is the first step in effectively managing those emotions.

Practice Mindfulness or Meditation: These practices can help you stay grounded and present, making it easier to handle emotions as they come up.

Engage in Physical Activity: Exercise can be a great way to release pent-up emotions and reduce stress. Even a short walk or some stretching can help.

Applying this to the real world: For instance, if you know you tend to feel anxious before tests, you could develop a pre-test routine that includes techniques like guided imagery or progressive muscle relaxation to help you manage your anxiety. By having a set of strategies ready, you can feel more prepared and less at the mercy of your emotions when triggers arise.

Use a Trigger Journal

A practical tool to boost your emotional intelligence, especially regarding triggers, is a trigger journal. This is different from an emotion log, which records your daily feelings and moods. In a trigger journal, you specifically document each instance when you feel a strong emotional response. Note down:

What Happened: Describe the event or situation that triggered your emotions.

How You Felt: Detail the emotions you experienced.

What You Thought: Capture the thoughts running through your mind at that moment.

How You Reacted: Write about your immediate reaction or response to the situation.

Over time, this journal will help you identify patterns in your emotional triggers and understand which strategies work best for you in managing your responses. Remember, the goal isn't to suppress your feelings but to manage them in a way that supports your well-being and helps you achieve your personal goals.

1.6 The Science of Stress and Its Impact on You

Stress is a universal experience, yet its impact is profoundly personal, often misunderstood until it manifests in ways that can no longer be ignored. In our bodies, stress initiates a complex cascade of physiological responses, beginning with the release of adrenaline and cortisol.

These hormones are your body's call to arms. Adrenaline increases your heart rate, elevates your blood pressure, and boosts energy supplies, while cortisol, the primary stress hormone, increases sugars in the bloodstream and enhances your brain's use of glucose. This hormonal surge is part of the fight-or-flight response that prepares you to face an immediate threat. However, when these hormones flood your system frequently—due to chronic stress—they can lead to significant health issues, both physical and mental.

The long-term effects of sustained high cortisol levels are particularly concerning. Physically, chronic stress can lead to cardiovascular problems such as high blood pressure and heart disease, as well as other issues like headaches, severe fatigue, and diabetes. Mentally, the picture is equally grim. Continuous exposure to stress can alter the brain's structure and function, leading to an increased risk of anxiety disorders and depression.

This is particularly critical to monitor during the teenage years, which is a pivotal time for brain development. The hippocampus, an area of the brain that regulates emotions and memory, can decrease in size under persistent stress, leading to difficulties in learning and memory retention and an increased risk of developing mood disorders.

Everyday Stress Triggers for Teens

- School pressure (tests, grades, college applications)
- Relationship drama (friends, dating, family conflicts)
- Body image concerns
- Social media stress (FOMO, cyberbullying, comparison trap)
- Uncertainty about the future
- Overscheduling and lack of downtime
- World events and societal pressures

Sound familiar? You're not alone. These are super common stressors for teens.

Stress-Busting Strategies

1. Time Management

- Use a planner or digital calendar to keep track of deadlines and commitments.
- Break big tasks into smaller, manageable chunks.
- Learn to prioritize—not everything needs to be done right now.

2. The Power of "No"

- It's okay to say no to extra commitments if you're feeling overwhelmed.
- Set boundaries with friends and family about your time and energy.

3. Stress-Relief Toolkit

- Find healthy ways to blow off steam: Exercise, art, music, journaling.
- Practice relaxation techniques like deep breathing or progressive muscle relaxation.
- Try mindfulness meditation to stay grounded in the present moment.

4. Sleep Is Your Superpower

- Aim for eight to ten hours of sleep per night.
- Establish a relaxing bedtime routine.
- Limit screen time before bed (easier said than done).

5. Fuel Your Body Right

- Eat regular, balanced meals.
- Stay hydrated—your brain needs water to function at its best.
- Limit caffeine and sugar, which can increase anxiety.

6. Connect and Share

- Talk to friends, family, or a counselor about what's stressing you out.
- Sometimes, just venting can make you feel better.

7. Reframe Your Thoughts

- Challenge negative self-talk. Instead of "I can't handle this," try "This is tough, but I can get through it."
- Look for the opportunity in challenges. What can you learn from this stressful situation?

8. Take Regular Breaks

- Schedule short breaks during study sessions or extended projects.
- Use this time to stretch, move around, or do something you enjoy.

9. Limit Social Media

- Set boundaries on your social media use.
- Remember, what you see online isn't always reality.

10. Celebrate Small Wins

- Acknowledge your accomplishments, no matter how small.
- This builds confidence and resilience in the face of stress.

Some stress is normal and even helpful. The key is learning to manage it so it doesn't manage you. If you're feeling overwhelmed by stress, don't hesitate to reach out for help. Your teachers, school counselors, or a mental health professional can provide additional support and strategies.

1.7 Emotions in the Digital Age: Social Media's Role

In today's world, where digital connections often outnumber face-to-face interactions, understanding the role of social media in our emotional lives is more crucial than ever. For many teens, platforms like Instagram, Snapchat, and TikTok aren't just apps but integral parts of daily life. While staying connected has its benefits, this constant connectivity can amplify feelings of loneliness, jealousy, and anxiety.

The curated perfection seen on social media profiles can lead to unhealthy comparisons, making your own life seem dull or inadequate. This digital showcase often skews reality, creating an environment where everyone else appears happier, more successful, or more attractive, fostering feelings of inadequacy and dissatisfaction.

However, it's not all negative. Social media can also have many positive impacts on emotional well-being. It can be a powerful tool for staying connected with friends and family, especially those who are not physically nearby. It allows for sharing experiences and building supportive communities. Many people find solace and understanding by joining groups or following pages that align with their interests or challenges. These communities can provide a sense of belonging and support, offering a place to share experiences, seek advice, and find companionship during times of stress or isolation.

Setting boundaries is key to maintaining a healthy relationship with social media.

Recognize when online interactions start replacing face-to-face connections or when scrolling through feeds becomes a compulsive habit. Implement designated "digital detox" times, such as setting aside specific times of day when screens are off-limits, like during meals or before bed. Being mindful of your consumption involves limiting the time spent online and critically evaluating your content. Ask yourself: Does this make me feel good about myself? Does it add value to my day? Encouraging these habits helps cultivate a more balanced and controlled digital life.

The impact of social media on self-esteem cannot be understated. It often presents unrealistic standards of beauty and success that can damage one's self-image. To combat this, it's important to foster a strong sense of self-worth independent of online likes or followers. Focus on your personal achievements and qualities rather than appearance, practice gratitude for what makes you unique, and engage in activities that boost confidence and bring real-world satisfaction. Curate your social media feeds to include positive influences and sources that uplift your mood and self-esteem, transforming your digital environment into a supportive resource.

Navigating the complex emotions elicited by our digital engagements is an essential skill in today's world. By understanding the dual impact of social media, setting healthy boundaries, and fostering a robust sense of self, you can harness these platforms to enhance, rather than undermine, your emotional well-being. As we continue to live more in the digital realm, remember that the power to shape that experience into a positive one lies with you. Embrace connectivity, explore communities, and use the tools to build a digital presence that reflects and supports who you are and aspire to be.

Strategies for Healthy Online Engagement

Managing healthy online communication and engagement is critical. Here are some practical strategies:

Set Boundaries: Limit your social media time using app timers or designated "phone-free" hours. For example, try a "no phones at the dinner table" rule or avoid social media for the first hour after waking up.

Curate Your Feed: Follow accounts that inspire and uplift you. Unfollow or mute those that consistently make you feel bad. Remember, it's your feed—you control what you see.

Reality Check: Remind yourself that social media isn't real life. People usually share their best moments, not their mundane or difficult times. Develop a healthy skepticism about what you see online.

Engage Mindfully: Before posting, ask yourself why you're sharing. Is it for yourself or for others' approval? Focus on sharing authentic experiences rather than seeking validation.

Take Breaks: Regular "digital detoxes" can help reset your relationship with social media. Start with small breaks, like a social media-free weekend, and see how it affects your mood and stress levels.

Focus on Real Connections: Prioritize face-to-face interactions and deep conversations over surface-level online interactions. Use social media to enhance real-life relationships, not replace them.

Practice Gratitude: Instead of comparing your life to others, focus on what you're grateful for in your own life. Consider starting a gratitude journal to shift your focus from what you lack to what you have.

Be a Critical Consumer: Develop media literacy skills. Question the sources of information you see online and fact-check before sharing or believing sensational news.

Use Privacy Settings: Protect your personal information and be mindful of what you share publicly. Once something is online, it can be hard to remove it completely.

Seek Balance: Use social media for connection and inspiration, but do not make it your only source of social interaction or self-esteem.

Dealing with Cyberbullying and Online Conflicts

Document Everything: Take screenshots of harmful messages or posts. This can be useful if you need to report the behavior to school authorities or social media platforms.

Don't Engage: Responding often escalates the situation. Block and report instead. Remember, you don't have to attend every argument you're invited to.

Seek Support: Talk to trusted friends, family, or school counselors about what's happening. You don't have to face this alone.

Know Your Rights: Many schools and platforms have policies against cyberbullying. Familiarize yourself with these and report violations.

Protect Your Privacy: Be cautious about what personal information you share online. The less ammunition bullies have, the better.

Build a Positive Online Presence: Engage in positive online activities and communities. This can help counteract negative experiences and provide a support network.

Practice Self-Care: Dealing with online negativity can be draining. Take care of your mental health through relaxation techniques, hobbies, and offline social support.

Remember, your worth isn't determined by your follower count or like tally. Use social media as a tool for connection and inspiration, not as a measure of your value.

In this chapter, we've explored the complex world of emotions and how they affect our daily lives. We've learned that emotions are more than just feelings - they're messages from our body and mind that help us understand what's going on around us. We've discovered how to recognize different emotions, understand where they come from, and manage them better. We've also looked at how stress impacts us and how social media can influence our feelings.

Remember, everyone experiences emotions differently, and that's okay. The goal isn't to get rid of emotions but to understand them better so we can handle life's ups and downs more easily. By paying attention to your feelings, using the strategies we've discussed, and being kind to yourself, you can develop stronger emotional intelligence and live a more balanced life.

Chapter 2
Building Emotional Resilience

Imagine you're playing a challenging level in a video game. Each time you face and overcome a challenge, you get better at the game and learn strategies that make you more adept for future levels. This is what resilience in real life looks like facing challenges, learning from them, and emerging stronger.

Resilience isn't about avoiding difficulties or emotions but developing the skills to tackle them head-on and bounce back with greater strength. In this chapter, we'll explore how building emotional resilience can fundamentally transform your approach to daily stressors and setbacks, helping you survive and thrive.

2.1 The Role of Resilience in Emotional Health

Resilience is often portrayed as harsh or enduring pain, but it's much more than simple emotional endurance or a stoic ability to absorb stress. At its core, resilience is about flexibility and adaptability. It's navigating through challenges, learning from them, and using that knowledge to cope more effectively with future problems.

Resilience involves a dynamic interaction between your characteristics and your environment, all shaped by experiences that foster a sense of competence and a belief in one's abilities. By understanding resilience in this way, you can see it not as a static trait you either have or don't have but as a set of skills you can develop and strengthen over time.

Resilience and Emotional Regulation

One critical benefit of resilience is its role in emotional regulation—the ability to manage and respond appropriately to an emotional experience.

Resilient individuals recognize when a particular emotion isn't serving them well and can adjust their response accordingly. For instance, if frustration at a homework assignment escalates to a point where it's hindering progress, a resilient teen might recognize this escalation and take a break, channeling their emotions into a different activity or changing their approach to the task to curb feelings of frustration.

This capacity to redirect your emotions can prevent them

from escalating into more intense feelings like anger or despair, thereby maintaining your emotional equilibrium.

Long-term Benefits of Resilience

Developing resilience in life offers profound long-term benefits for your mental health. Studies have shown that resilient individuals are less likely to suffer from conditions like depression and anxiety. Instead, they often experience greater well-being and satisfaction in life.

This isn't because resilient individuals experience fewer difficulties. Instead, they possess skills and a mindset that enable them to deal with challenges more effectively. Resilience provides a buffer against the types of stressors that can lead to mental health disorders and fosters a proactive approach to tackling life's challenges head-on.

Cultivating a Resilience Mindset

Building a resilience mindset is all about changing how you see and react to challenges. Instead of viewing obstacles as setbacks, start seeing them as opportunities to grow. Each challenge is a chance to learn something new about yourself and sharpen your problem-solving skills. This isn't just about being optimistic. It's about recognizing the potential for personal growth in every tough situation.

Action Plan to Build Resilience

Shift Your Perspective

Daily Challenges as Growth Opportunities: Whenever you face a problem, remind yourself it's a chance to learn and grow.

Embrace Learning: Focus on what you can learn from each experience rather than the negative aspects.

Strengthen Your Support Network

Connect with Friends and Family: Regularly reach out to those who care about you.

Join Supportive Communities: Engage in groups or activities that provide a sense of belonging and support.

Set Realistic Goals and Expectations

Break Down Goals: Divide large goals into smaller, manageable steps.

Celebrate Small Wins: Acknowledge and celebrate progress, no matter how small.

Develop Positive Coping Strategies

Exercise Regularly: Physical activity can boost your mood and reduce stress.

Practice Mindfulness: Techniques like meditation or deep breathing can help keep you grounded.

Engage in Hobbies: Spend time doing things you enjoy to relax and recharge.

Keep a Resilience Journal

Document Daily Challenges: Write down what happened, how you felt, and how you responded.

Reflect on Learning: Note what you learned from each challenge and how you can apply it in the future.

Track Your Growth: Over time, review your entries to see how your resilience has improved.

Building resilience is an ongoing journey. It requires commitment and practice, but the benefits—better emotional regulation, reduced risk of mental health issues, and a more fulfilling life—are worth the effort. Every challenge you face is an opportunity to become more skilled at navigating life's complexities. Keep working on these strategies, and you'll find yourself more capable and confident in handling whatever comes your way.

In this chapter, we've explored the vital role of resilience in our emotional health and overall well-being. We've learned that resilience isn't about toughing it out or avoiding challenges—it's about developing the flexibility to adapt and grow from life's ups and downs. Remember, resilience is a skill that can be cultivated over time, not a fixed trait you either have or don't. By shifting our perspective to see challenges as opportunities for growth, strengthening our support networks, setting realistic goals, and developing positive coping strategies, we can build our resilience muscle.

The journey to becoming more resilient might not always be easy, but the rewards are immense—better emotional regulation, improved mental health, and a more fulfilling life. As you move forward, keep in mind that every challenge you face is a chance to become stronger and more capable. With practice and patience, you'll find yourself better equipped to navigate life's complexities and bounce back from setbacks with greater ease and confidence.

Chapter 3
Tools for Emotional Regulation

I magine sitting in your favorite spot, a cozy corner of your room, or a quiet park bench. Suddenly, your phone vibrates—a message pops up, and it's not good news: Your heart races, your stomach churns, and your mind whirls. Now, imagine being able to calm this storm instantly within you, almost like you have a remote control for your emotions. This isn't just a fanciful idea. It's entirely possible with mindfulness meditation.

In this chapter, we will delve into mindfulness, a powerful tool that can transform your approach to life's ups and downs, enhancing your focus, resilience, and overall well-being.

3.1 Mastering Mindfulness: A Teen's Guide

Introduction to Mindfulness Meditation

Mindfulness meditation is an ancient practice, but its benefits are timeless and particularly relevant in today's fast-paced world of constant distractions. At its core, mindfulness is about being fully present in the moment, aware of where we are and what we're doing, without being overly reactive or overwhelmed by what's happening around us. It teaches you to focus on your thoughts, feelings, bodily sensations, and surrounding environment to increase your awareness and clarity.

One of mindfulness meditation's primary advantages is its ability to reduce stress. It also enhances concentration, supports emotional regulation, and bolsters resilience, making it an essential tool for anyone, especially teenagers, navigating the complexities of modern life.

Step-by-step Guide to Mindfulness Meditation

Starting a mindfulness meditation practice might initially seem daunting, but it can be simple. Here's a beginner-friendly guide to get you started:

- **Find a Quiet Space:** Choose a calm and quiet place where you won't be disturbed.
- **Set a Time Limit:** If you're beginning, choose a short time, such as five or ten minutes.

- **Get Comfortable:** Sit on a chair or the floor with your head, neck, and back straight but not stiff.
- **Focus on Your Breath**: Pay attention to the sensation of breath entering and leaving your nostril or how your belly rises and falls.
- **Return to Breathing:** Your mind will wander. This is normal. As soon as you notice your mind wandering, gently return your focus to your breath.

Common Challenges and How to Overcome Them

It's usual for beginners to face challenges such as wandering thoughts or physical discomfort when attempting to incorporate a mindfulness program. These obstacles can be frustrating, but they're part of the process. When you notice your mind wandering, gently bring it back to your breath—this is mindfulness practice. If you encounter physical discomfort, adjust your posture or sit position. Sometimes, the discomfort is part of meditation, teaching you about acceptance and pliability.

Mindfulness Meditation and the Brain

Scientific research has shown that mindfulness meditation can significantly benefit the brain. MRI scans have observed brain structure and activity changes both during and after meditation. Regular meditation practice can increase the density of gray matter in brain regions linked to learning, memory, emotion regulation, and empathy. Additionally, mindfulness meditation decreases activity in the amygdala, the part of the brain responsible for processing stress and fear, which correlates with reduced stress levels.

These changes in the brain improve cognitive and emotional skills and enhance your ability to handle stress, maintain focus, and recover from adverse events more quickly. Integrating mindfulness into your daily routine can be a game-changer, helping you navigate the challenges of your teenage life with greater calm and clarity. By learning to focus your attention and become more aware of your thoughts and feelings, you will gain a powerful tool that can improve your emotional and mental well-being in lasting ways.

3.2 Visualization Techniques for Stress Reduction

Imagine you have the power to instantly transport yourself to a serene beach with waves gently lapping at the shore or see yourself acing an upcoming test with confidence—this is the essence of visualization.

Visualization, or mental imagery, is a powerful psychological strategy that involves creating vivid, detailed images in your mind, serving as a mental escape to stress relief and clarity. This technique leverages the brain's inability to distinguish between real and vividly imagined experiences, thus providing emotional and physiological benefits similar to actual experiences.

Visualization can be a potent tool for managing stress and achieving mental clarity. By mentally simulating positive outcomes or calming environments, you can invoke physical and emotional responses that parallel real-life interactions. For instance, visualizing a peaceful setting can trigger relaxation responses in the body, such as reduced heart rate and lower blood pressure, like what you would experience if you were in that tranquil place.

This makes visualization an excellent tool for managing stress and preparing for upcoming challenges by envisioning successful outcomes, which can boost confidence and reduce anxiety.

Guided Visualization Exercises

To begin with visualization, try these scripted exercises designed to promote relaxation and mental clarity:

Peaceful Place Visualization: Close your eyes and imagine where you feel completely at ease. This could be a quiet forest, a sunny beach, or a cozy room. Visualize the details of this place—the sounds, the smells, and how it feels. See yourself in this place, feeling calm and relaxed. Spend a few minutes enjoying the sensation of peace that this place brings you.

Success Visualization: Think of an upcoming event where you want to succeed, such as a presentation or a sports match. Picture yourself performing perfectly: Imagine looking confident, feeling prepared, and executing every part of the task flawlessly. Focus on the positive emotions you feel and the reactions of others around you. This exercise can help build your confidence and reduce anxiety about the event.

Tailoring Visualization to Personal Needs

To make visualization more effective, personalize your scenarios to address specific stressors or goals. Start by identifying what you feel anxious or stressed about, then create images that counteract these feelings. For example, if you are nervous about an upcoming test, visualize yourself calmly reviewing the questions and confidently writing down the answers. Regularly practicing these personalized visualizations allows you to feel more in control of your emotions and more confident about handling stressful situations.

Integrating Visualization with Mindfulness

Combining visualization with mindfulness techniques can enhance the benefits of both practices. Start your visualization with a mindfulness exercise, such as focusing on your breath or conducting a body scan—focusing on each part of your body and taking a mental inventory of how it feels. This helps center your mind and prepares you for visualization.

After completing your visualization, return to a state of mindfulness, focusing again on your breath or the physical sensations in your body. This combination can help deepen your relaxation and reinforce the positive effects of both practices.

Visualization is not just a technique but a skill that improves with practice. The more vividly and frequently you can imagine these calming or successful scenarios, the more natural and effective they will become. Visualization offers a portable and powerful way to enhance your mental and emotional well-being, whether to calm down before a big game, prepare for an oral presentation, or find peace within the parameters of a hectic day.

As you continue to explore and refine your visualization skills, remember that the clarity and tranquility you wish to achieve are fleeting moments of escape and stepping stones to greater emotional resilience and clarity.

3.3 Mindfulness Exercises for Different Settings

Mindfulness isn't just reserved for quiet moments alone. It can be woven into the fabric of your everyday activities, turning routine actions into opportunities for growth and self-awareness. Integrating mindfulness into daily activities can transform even the most mundane tasks into calm and clear moments, enhancing your mental focus and emotional balance.

Mindfulness in Daily Activities

Let's start with something as simple as eating, an activity we often complete on autopilot. Next time you have a meal, try engaging fully with the experience. Notice the color, texture, and aroma of your food. Chew slowly, savoring each bite, and pay attention to the flavors and sensations in your mouth. This practice, known as mindful eating, enhances your dining experience and can improve internal functions like digestion. It can also signal when you are full, preventing overeating.

Walking, another mindless everyday activity, also offers a perfect opportunity for mindfulness. Instead of rushing to your destination with your mind on other things, slow down and notice each step. Feel your feet touch the ground, the rhythm of your pace, and how your arms swing with each stride. Observe the sights and sounds around you, and perhaps the warmth of the sun or the breeze against your skin. This act of mindful walking can transform a simple commute into a refreshing break, clearing your mind and relieving stress.

Listening to music provides yet another avenue for practicing mindfulness. Instead of letting music be just background noise, challenge yourself to actually listen. Focus on the lyrics, the melody, and the instruments. Identify each sound and how they combine to create the whole piece. This deep engagement with the music can help you feel more connected and present, providing a mental break from your daily worries.

Mindfulness at School

School can be a hotbed of stress, but mindfulness can help you navigate this environment more effectively. Before a test or a presentation, take a few minutes to practice mindful breathing. Close your eyes, breathe deeply, and focus solely on the rhythm of your inhalation and exhalation.

This can help ease your nerves, center your thoughts, and improve your concentration. During transitions, instead of rushing immediately to the next class or checking your phone, take a moment to reflect on what you just learned and set an intention for the next class. This brief moment of mindfulness can help you stay grounded and focused throughout the school day.

Mindfulness in Nature

Spending time in nature is a beautiful way to practice mindfulness and reconnect with the environment. Try a mindful walk in a park or any natural setting. Engage all your senses —notice the colors of the leaves, the patterns of light and shadow, the sounds of birds or rustling leaves, and the smell of the earth. Each step can help you feel more rooted in the world around you, enhancing your well-being and providing a peaceful retreat from daily stresses.

Mindfulness for Emotional Regulation

Mindfulness can be particularly effective for managing intense emotions. When you feel anger or frustration bubbling up, mindful breathing can quickly and effectively regain control. Pause, take a deep breath, and focus on breathing slowly and deeply.

This can help deactivate the body's stress response and allow you to approach the situation more clearly. Another technique is to observe your emotions without judgment—acknowledge them and understand they are temporary and do not define you. This detachment allows you to choose how to respond rather than react impulsively.

Incorporating mindfulness into various settings and activities enhances your ability to focus and perform tasks more efficiently and improves emotional resilience. Whether through mindful eating, walking, listening to music, or breathing exercises, each moment of mindfulness adds up, helping you build a stronger, more aware, and emotionally balanced self. As you continue to practice these techniques, mindfulness becomes a natural part of your daily routine, enriching your experiences and interactions in all aspects of life.

3.4 Creating a Personal Meditation Routine

Getting into a meditation routine is like starting a new adventure that's all about you. Here's how to make it work for your needs and goals:

Identify Your Goals

- **Look Inside**: Think about why you want to meditate. Is it to reduce school stress or social anxiety? Boost your concentration for better grades? Sleep better at night?
- **Set Expectations**: Understand what you hope

to get out of it. This will help shape how you meditate.

- **Make It a Daily Habit**
- **Start Small**: Even a few minutes a day can make a big difference. Begin with short sessions and gradually increase the time.
- **Find Your Time**: Pick a time when you won't be interrupted. Morning meditation can set a calm tone for the day, while evening sessions can help you unwind.
- **Be Consistent**: Just like brushing your teeth or eating breakfast, make meditation a regular part of your routine. Consistency is key to seeing benefits.

Create a Meditation Space

- **Choose a Spot**: Find a quiet corner of your room where you can relax without distractions.
- **Make It Inviting**: Add a soft blanket, a few pillows, or a plant to make the space cozy. Keep it tidy and peaceful.
- **Manage Noise**: If you're easily distracted by noise, use soothing background music or a white noise app to help you focus.

Track Your Progress

- **Keep a Journal or Use an App**: Write down

your thoughts and feelings after each session. Note what works and what doesn't.

- **Review Regularly**: Look back over your entries to see how you've improved. Noticing changes in your focus and stress levels can be really motivating.

Adapt as You Grow

- **Regular Check-ins**: As you get better at meditating, your goals might change. Adjust your practice accordingly.
- **Explore New Techniques**: Try extending your meditation time, experimenting with different methods, or focusing on new areas like gratitude or empathy.

Meditation is an ever-evolving practice that grows with you. By keeping it flexible and tailored to your needs, you'll find it easier to navigate life's ups and downs with a calm and focused mind.

3.5 Breathing Techniques for Instant Calm

Breathing is the most natural thing we do, and we usually don't even think about it. But did you know that by changing how you breathe, you can have a huge impact on your mental and physical state? It's true! Controlled breathing exercises can help you relax, calm your mind, and reduce stress and anxiety. Here's how it works.

When you practice controlled breathing, you engage your parasympathetic nervous system. This system, often called the "rest and digest" system, plays a crucial role in regulating your body's unconscious actions. Unlike the "fight or flight" response managed by the sympathetic nervous system, which prepares your body to deal with immediate threats, the parasympathetic nervous system promotes a state of calm and relaxation.

The parasympathetic nervous system is responsible for slowing down your heart rate and lowering blood pressure. When activated, it helps your body conserve energy by slowing the heart rate, increasing intestinal and gland activity, and relaxing sphincter muscles in the gastrointestinal tract. This creates a feeling of calm and relaxation, counteracting the stress response.

Breathing Techniques

Let's get into some specific breathing techniques that you can use to find immediate relief when stress levels start to rise. One effective method is **diaphragmatic breathing**, also known as belly breathing. To do this, you breathe deeply into your belly, allowing your diaphragm to do the work, which helps your lungs to fully expand. The technique is simple: Place one hand on your belly and the other on your chest. As you breathe in slowly through your nose, you should feel your belly rise, and the hand on it should increase more than the one on your chest. This encourages full oxygen exchange and can immediately reduce your heartbeat rate and lower or stabilize your blood pressure, providing a sense of calm.

Another powerful technique is the **4-7-8 breathing method** previously mentioned, which involves breathing in for four seconds, holding the breath for seven seconds, and exhaling for eight seconds. This method is perfect for reducing anxiety or helping to induce sleep. By forcing the rhythm of your breathing, you enhance the effects of diaphragmatic breathing, further stimulating your parasympathetic nervous system and enhancing your calm.

Alternate nostril breathing, a standard yoga practice, is another technique that promotes calm and improves focus. Here's how you do it:

1. Close your right nostril with your right thumb and inhale slowly through your left nostril.
2. Close your left nostril with your fingers, open your right nostril, and exhale slowly.
3. Reverse the process by inhaling through the right nostril and exhaling through the left.

This technique calms and centers the mind, enhances cardiovascular function, and lowers stress levels.

Practice Scenarios

Knowing these techniques is one thing, but applying them in real-life scenarios is where they truly make a difference. You're about to enter an exam room, and the nerves kick in. This is a perfect moment for 4-7-8 breathing. By controlling your breath this way, you can calm your nervous system, clear your mind, and focus on the task immediately in front of you. Or perhaps you're in a heated discussion with a friend or family member. This might be a good time to step back and engage in diaphragmatic breathing, which can help you maintain your composure and handle the situation more thoughtfully.

Creating a Habit of Breathing Exercises

To truly benefit from these breathing exercises, you should start by making them a part of your daily routine. It can be as simple as practicing diaphragmatic breathing for a few minutes each morning when you wake up or using the 4-7-8 technique each night before you go to sleep. You can also link these practices to daily activities as reminders. For instance, practice a few rounds of alternate nostril breathing while waiting for your morning coffee to brew or during a break between classes. By associating breathing exercises with regular activities, you'll be more likely to remember and commit to practicing them, making it easier to access these techniques when needed.

Breathing exercises offer a simple, quick, and effective way to manage your emotions and reduce stress, enhancing your overall well-being. As you continue to practice these techniques, you might find that not only are you able to calm yourself more quickly and effectively, but you're also culti-vating a greater sense of control over your emotional life, empowering you to face each day with confidence and clarity—so inhale, exhale, and see what all you can accomplish when you focus on your breath.

3.6 The Role of Physical Exercise in Emotional Health

Engaging in physical activity isn't just about keeping your body fit. It's also a powerful way to enhance your emotional and mental health. When you exercise, your body releases chemicals called endorphins—often known as "feel-good" hormones—which act as natural painkillers and mood elevators.

Regular physical activity can help alleviate symptoms of depression and anxiety by promoting changes in the parts of the brain that regulate stress and anxiety.

Moreover, exercise helps boost your overall mood by producing endorphins, which can make problems seem more manageable, and reducing feelings of loneliness and isolation by connecting you with others in a fun and relaxed setting.

Physical Activities

Let's explore various physical activities that are particularly effective for emotional regulation. Yoga, for instance, combines physical postures, breathing exercises, and meditation to enhance mindful awareness and relaxation. Regular yoga practice can decrease the body's stress responses and reduce heart rate, all while lowering blood pressure and easing respiration.

Another beneficial activity is running, which can help clear your mind and reduce stress. The rhythmic, pounding beat of your feet on the pavement can be meditative, relieving tension and anxiety.

A third activity, dancing, is another powerful exercise that allows you to express yourself creatively, which can be incredibly therapeutic. Dancing involves cardiovascular conditioning, strength, balance, and coordination, providing a full-body workout that is fun and energizing.

Finally, participating in team sports supports physical fitness. It improves your mood and mental health by providing social interactions which aids in reducing feelings of isolation, and boosting your confidence as part of a team.

Daily Integration

Integrating physical activity into your daily routine might seem challenging, especially when balancing things like schoolwork, social life, and family obligations. However, the key is not to view exercise as "just another chore" but as an enjoyable part of your day.

Begin by first identifying a few physical activities you enjoy, for example: A dance class, a morning jog, or a casual basketball game with friends. Aim for consistency rather than intensity. Even twenty minutes of physical activity can have significant health benefits.

Try to incorporate exercise into your daily activities—things like biking to school, taking the stairs instead of the elevator, or taking a walk while talking on the phone can help you get a few more physical moments throughout your day with a small impact on your schedule. These small changes can add up, making exercise a natural part of your life without overwhelming your schedule.

Overcoming Obstacles

Even though physical activity has clear benefits, facing challenges like needing more time, motivation, or resources is normal. Overcoming these obstacles is crucial for building and maintaining an active lifestyle. If you're short on time, try to fit exercise into your daily routine, like walking or biking to school. If motivation is your issue, set realistic goals and find a workout buddy to keep you accountable.

For other barriers, like not having access to a gym, use online workout videos or apps that offer exercises you can do at home with little or no equipment. The key is to find what works for you and make it a part of your everyday life.

Physical exercise offers a range of psychological benefits, from improving mood and reducing symptoms of depression and anxiety to enhancing self-esteem and cognitive function. You can harness these benefits by finding physical activities you enjoy and integrating them into your daily routine, leading to improved emotional health and a more balanced life.

As you continue to explore and engage in different forms of physical exercise, remember that every step, stretch, or dance move is a step toward physical health and emotional well-being.

3.7 Nutrition and Mood: Foods That Affect Feelings

Ever notice how a hearty breakfast can set you up for a great day while skipping a meal can leave you irritable and unfocused? It's not just about filling your stomach—what you eat can significantly affect your mood and mental health.

This is largely due to the gut-brain axis, a complex network linking your gastrointestinal tract and brain. Your gut is home to countless bacteria that play a crucial role in producing neurotransmitters like serotonin, which is primarily found in the intestines and is essential for mood regulation. This means the health of your gut can directly influence your brain's function and your emotional state.

Nutritional Building Blocks

As you begin to understand this connection, it becomes clear why maintaining a diet that supports gut health is vital for emotional well-being. Foods rich in omega-3 fatty acids, such as salmon, flaxseeds, and walnuts, enhance brain function and mood. These fats are crucial components of brain cells, enhancing their ability to communicate effectively. Whole grains like oats and brown rice are also essential, as they slowly release glucose into your bloodstream, providing a steady energy level that helps stabilize your mood.

Lean proteins, including chicken, tofu, and legumes, contain amino acids, which are the building blocks for neurotransmitters in the brain, affecting how you feel and react to situations. Additionally, a diverse array of fruits and vegetables provides vitamins, minerals, and antioxidants that combat inflammation, which has been linked to depression and anxiety.

However, just as some foods can uplift your mood, others might drag it down. High sugar intake, for example, can cause a surge in blood glucose levels followed by a sharp drop, leading to mood swings and energy slumps.

Similarly, excessive caffeine can disrupt your sleep patterns and increase anxiety levels, while junk food, often high in fats and sugars, can exacerbate feelings of depression and fatigue. Understanding these physiological impacts can help you make more informed choices about what you eat, especially in times of stress or when you need a mental boost.

Create a Plan

Creating a balanced diet plan doesn't have to be a chore or involve drastic changes. Start off small by incorporating mood-enhancing foods into your meals, ensuring you get a good mix of proteins, fats, and carbohydrates at each meal to keep your energy and mood levels stable.

For instance, a breakfast of eggs (rich in protein and fat) with whole-grain toast (a good source of fiber and slow-releasing carbohydrates) can provide a solid start to the day. Snacking on fruits and nuts instead of chips or candy can also significantly affect how you feel throughout the day.

When dining out, opt to order dishes with balanced nutrients and be mindful of portion sizes, as overeating can lead to discomfort and lethargy.

Nutrition Labels

Learning to read nutrition labels is another skill that can help you make better food choices. Look for products low in added sugars and high in fiber and protein. As you grow, learning to cook simple, healthy meals at home can also be a fun and rewarding way to take control of your diet and mood.

Start with simple recipes incorporating fresh ingredients and experiment with herbs and spices to add flavor without extra calories or sodium.

Understanding nutrition's critical role in emotional health and making mindful choices about what you eat can significantly influence your mood and overall well-being. As you continue to explore the impact of different foods on your emotions, remember that small, consistent changes can have a profound effect, helping you feel more balanced and ready to tackle whatever comes your way.

3.8 The Importance of Sleep for Emotional Stability

Sleep is a core piece of the foundation that makes up your mental and emotional well-being, yet it's one of the first to be compromised during stressful times or when deadlines loom. Think about how irritability creeps in when you've skipped a few hours of sleep or how overwhelming challenges seem when you're running low on rest. This isn't just about feeling tired.

Sleep deprivation significantly affects your ability to regulate emotions, making sadness, anger, and stress more intense and more challenging to manage. Without adequate sleep, your brain struggles to balance chemicals and hormones that affect mood and thoughts, which can enhance negative emotions and diminish the effectiveness of your coping strategies.

Good Sleep Hygiene

Developing good sleep hygiene is essential for maintaining emotional balance. It starts with setting a regular sleep schedule—going to bed and waking up at the same time every day (yes, even on weekends). This consistency reinforces your body's sleep-wake cycle and can help improve the quality of your sleep.

A Restful Environment

Creating a restful environment for sleep is also crucial. Make your bedroom ideal for sleeping. Keep it cool, quiet, and dark, and invest in a good-quality mattress and pillows. It's also wise to avoid stimulants like caffeine and nicotine close to bedtime, as they can disrupt your ability to fall asleep.

Similarly, while it might be tempting to scroll through social media or binge a few show episodes before bed, the blue light emitted by screens can inhibit the production of melatonin, the hormone that regulates sleep. Instead, develop a relaxing bedtime routine that might include reading a book, listening to soothing music, or practicing relaxation exercises to help signal to your body that it's time to wind down.

Common Sleep Issues

Addressing common sleep issues, specifically among teens, such as difficulty falling asleep, nighttime awakenings, or oversleeping, might require specific strategies. If you are tossing and turning, unable to drift away to dreamland, try keeping a sleep diary to identify any habits or activities contributing to your insomnia.

Establishing a pre-sleep routine that involves calming activities can also make a big difference. For those who wake up frequently during the night, it might help to look at environmental factors. Is your room too hot or too noisy? Adjusting these conditions might provide a solution.

And for those who tend to oversleep, it's essential to get to the root of why this is happening—is it due to a lack of quality sleep or perhaps a way of escaping stress? Understanding the cause can help find the right approach.

Benefits of Napping

Everyone loves a good nap, right? You'll be happy to know that naps can also be beneficial in maintaining alertness and emotional balance, especially when nighttime sleep isn't sufficient.

However, getting the timing and duration of naps right is essential to avoid interfering with your sleep cycle. A short nap of 20-30 minutes can be revitalizing without leaving you feeling groggy or affecting your ability to sleep at night. Try to schedule naps for the early afternoon, when there's a natural dip in your circadian rhythms, and avoid napping too late. Remember, while naps can be helpful to catch up on missed sleep, they shouldn't be used as a substitute for getting adequate sleep each night.

Understanding sleep's critical role in emotional regulation and implementing strategies to improve sleep quality and manage common sleep issues can significantly enhance your overall emotional strength and stability. Whether adjusting your environment to make it more conducive to rest, establishing routines that signal to your body it's time to wind down, or using naps strategically; these steps can lead to noticeable improvements in how you feel and interact with the world around you.

As you continue to explore and apply these practices, your sleep is improving, and your ability to handle daily life's emotional ups and downs is also becoming more robust.

3.9 Yoga for Stress and Anxiety Relief

As mentioned earlier, yoga, an ancient practice that marries physical postures, breathing exercises, and meditation, offers a holistic approach to mental health, particularly in easing stress, anxiety, and depression. Its benefits are rooted in physical wellness and fostering deeper connections with one's mental and emotional states. Yoga can significantly lower stress hormone levels, enhance mood, and improve emotional flexibility.

This is particularly relevant for teens, who often navigate high levels of school pressure and social anxiety. The mindful breathing and meditative aspects of yoga teach you to manage your response to stress, replacing impulsiveness and reactivity with thoughtful awareness and calmness.

Poses

Yoga introduces a variety of poses and breathing techniques that can help calm the mind and alleviate stress and anxiety. Basic postures like the Child's Pose can evoke a sense of physical and emotional security, soothing the nervous system. On the other hand, the Tree Pose promotes concentration and balance, drawing your focus away from worries and grounding you in the present.

Pair these poses with deep, controlled breathing, which helps reduce stress by slowing the heartbeat and lowering blood pressure, enhancing feelings of peace and stability.

Daily Incorporation

Incorporating yoga into your daily routine doesn't require a heavy commitment and can be adjusted to fit your lifestyle and preferences. Even short sessions of yoga can provide benefits. You might start with a few minutes each morning to help set a calm tone for the day or use it as a tool to unwind in the evening. Many schools offer yoga classes as part of their physical education programs for those new to the practice, providing a guided and supportive way to learn.

Alternatively, numerous apps and online platforms offer yoga sessions that range from beginner to advanced levels, making it easy to practice from home at your convenience. These digital options often include a variety of styles and lengths of practice, ensuring something fits everyone's needs and schedules.

Mindfulness and Meditation

You already know how important mindfulness is for your emotional health and coping strategies, but did you know mindfulness and meditation are integral parts of yoga that significantly enhance its stress-relieving benefits?

These practices encourage reflective awareness, helping you recognize and release internal tensions and anxieties. A yoga session typically ends with the Savasana or Corpse Pose, which involves lying flat on your back and entering a deep state of relaxation, allowing you to assimilate the physical and emotional benefits of the practice entirely. This mindful relaxation can teach you to observe your thoughts and emotions without judgment, leading to greater emotional awareness and stability. Over time, this practice can help you develop a more mindful approach to your daily life, enabling you to navigate stress and anxiety with more ease and resilience.

Integrating yoga into your life allows you to embrace a powerful tool that enhances your physical flexibility and strength and supports your mental health and emotional well-being. Whether through breathing exercises that calm the mind, postures that release physical tension, or meditative practices that foster inner peace, yoga offers a comprehensive approach to reducing stress and anxiety.

As you continue to explore and practice yoga, it becomes a vital part of your strategy for maintaining mental health and emotional balance, helping you manage the pressures of teenage life with grace and stability.

3.10 Creating Your Emotional Safety Plan

Navigating the ups and downs of your emotional landscape isn't just about managing day-to-day stress—it's also important to have strategies for those moments when emotions threaten to overwhelm you.

This is where an emotional safety plan comes into play. It acts as a personalized roadmap to guide you through acute emotional distress and prevent potential crises. Think of it as a customized emergency response plan for your mental health, tailored to offer support when you need it the most.

Emotional Safety

Emotional safety is a set of strategies you can turn to during distress. It works to outline practical steps that help stabilize your emotional state, preventing a challenging situation from escalating into something unmanageable.

The plan is unique to each person, crafted to fit your specific emotional triggers and preferred coping mechanisms. It typically includes identifying your warning signs—those first hints that your emotional state is beginning to decline. These signs might be physical (like a racing heart), emotional (feeling suddenly overwhelmed), or behavioral (withdrawing from friends). Recognizing these signs early on can prompt you to take steps to manage your emotions before they spiral.

The Core

The plan's core involves detailed coping strategies that effectively diffuse your emotional distress. These might include breathing exercises, listening to a specific playlist, or engaging in physical activity. It's about knowing what works for you and having these actions ready.

Additionally, the plan should include a list of people who can provide support when needed—whether it's a trusted friend, a family member, or a mental health professional. Sometimes, just talking to someone can give immense relief. Finally, identify environments where you feel safe and calm. These are places you can go to regain your composure, whether it's a favorite park bench or a cozy corner of your local library.

Customization

Customizing your emotional safety plan is critical because it must resonate with your personal experiences and preferences. Start by reflecting on the past when you felt overwhelmed and consider what helped (or would have helped) you regain control. Experiment with different strategies to find what genuinely enables you to feel better.

Remember, what works for one person might not work for another, and that's perfectly okay. The goal is to develop a plan that feels like a reliable safety net tailored just for you.

Plan Flexibility

It's also essential to keep your emotional safety plan dynamic. As you grow and change, so too will your emotional needs. Make it a habit to review and update your plan regularly—perhaps every few months or after any significant life event or change in your emotional health.

This ensures the plan evolves with you and continues to serve its purpose effectively. Regular reviews also allow you to reassess what's working and what isn't, allowing you to make necessary adjustments to support your emotional well-being better.

In crafting your emotional safety plan, you take an essential step toward self-care and resilience. By outlining clear steps to manage emotional highs and lows, you confidently empower yourself to face life's challenges. This plan becomes a personal toolkit, always at your disposal, to help navigate the complexities of emotions and stress. As you progress, remember that each step in your plan is toward a more stable, fulfilled, and emotionally healthy life. This proactive approach enhances your ability to cope with immediate stressors and contributes to long-term emotional resilience and well-being.

In this chapter, we've explored a wealth of techniques to enhance emotional well-being and resilience. From the calming practice of mindfulness meditation to the power of visualization, we've discovered ways to navigate life's challenges with greater ease. We've learned how to integrate mindfulness into daily activities, create personalized meditation routines, and use breathing techniques for instant calm. The importance of physical exercise, proper nutrition, and quality sleep in maintaining emotional health has been highlighted.

We've also explored yoga as a holistic approach to stress management and the value of creating an emotional safety plan for difficult times. By incorporating these practices into your life, you're building a toolkit for emotional resilience and overall well-being. Remember, developing these skills is a journey—be patient with yourself and celebrate your progress along the way. With consistent practice, you'll find yourself better equipped to handle stress, regulate your emotions, and cultivate a deeper sense of inner peace.

Chapter 4
Communication and Emotional Expression

Imagine standing at a crossroads, with each direction leading to a different way of expressing your thoughts and feelings. One path might be the aggressive route, where voices are raised, and words can sting. Another path could be passive, where you say little and hide your true feelings.

Consider the middle path of assertiveness, where communication is open, honest, and respectful. This is the path we'll explore in this chapter. Learning to be assertive is like discovering a voice you didn't know you had. It's about speaking your reality without offending others or losing your self-respect. We'll dive into what being assertive means, why it's important, and how you can master this vital skill to improve your relationships and navigate your emotional world.

4.1 Assertiveness Training: Speak Up Without Fighting

Understanding Assertiveness

Assertiveness is the quality of being self-assured and confident without being aggressive. In a world where the loudest voices often dominate, assertiveness is your tool for being heard over the noise without having to shout. It's about respecting your own needs and feelings and those of others.

Unlike aggression, which imposes your views on others, or passivity, which silences your voice, assertiveness finds a balance. It involves expressing your thoughts and feelings openly and honestly while also considering the rights and views of others. This balanced approach fosters healthy relationships built on mutual respect and understanding.

One of the key benefits of being assertive is that it helps you handle conflicts more effectively and maintain healthier relationships. When you communicate assertively, you directly address issues as they arise, preventing misunderstandings and resentments from building up. This doesn't just apply to negative feelings. Being assertive means sharing positive feelings more freely.

By cultivating assertiveness, you empower yourself to negotiate, refuse when necessary, and ask for what you need—all essential skills as you navigate the challenges of teenage life and beyond.

Techniques for Assertive Communication

Mastering assertive communication involves using specific phrases and techniques that promote clear and respectful interaction. One fundamental technique is using "I" statements, which allow you to express your feelings and thoughts without blaming or accusing others.

For example, instead of saying, "You never listen to me," try, "I feel upset when I feel like I'm not being heard." This shift reduces the likelihood of the other person becoming defensive and keeps the focus on your experience.

Another technique is to maintain open body language—avoid crossing your arms or rolling your eyes, as these can send signals of aggression or disinterest. Keep your posture relaxed and open, make eye contact, and use a calm, steady tone of voice. These non-verbal cues reinforce the sincerity and respect central to assertive communication.

Role-playing Scenarios

Practicing assertiveness can be done through role-playing exercises, which provide a safe space to try out your responses to different scenarios. For instance, imagine you're faced with peer pressure to skip class.

A passive response might be following the plan despite your reservations. An aggressive response might involve lashing out angrily at your peers. An assertive response would be calmly stating, "I understand you want to skip class, but I'm uncomfortable. I'm going to stay."

Role-playing this kind of scenario with friends or family can help you feel more confident handling similar real-life situations.

Handling Responses to Assertiveness

Being assertive doesn't always lead to the outcome for which you might hope. Sometimes, it might provoke negative responses from others. Preparing for these possibilities is part of learning to be assertive.

If someone responds to your assertiveness with anger or aggression, it's essential to remain calm and not mirror their hostility. Continue to express your feelings and needs respectfully, and if the situation escalates, permit yourself to walk away. The goal is maintaining your dignity and respect, not winning an argument.

Communicating assertively is a powerful way to enhance emotional expression and develop stronger, healthier relationships. It allows you to navigate the complexities of social interactions and personal relationships with confidence and poise. As you practice these skills, you'll find that you're better able to express yourself and are more capable of handling the diverse and often challenging landscape of human emotions and relationships.

4.2 The Art of Saying No: Setting Boundaries

In your daily interactions, each relationship adds its own color and texture to your life, but what happens when these relationships become overwhelming, stretching you beyond your comfort zone? This is where setting boundaries becomes essential. Boundaries are invisible lines you draw around yourself to protect your energy, time, and emotional well-being. They help you define what you're comfortable with and how you want to be treated by others. This is crucial for maintaining your self-respect and personal integrity.

Boundary Lines

Think of boundaries as personal property lines that mark where your emotional and mental territory begins and ends. They help you manage stress and avoid burnout by clearly delineating what you can handle from yourself and others. For instance, setting a boundary around your time might mean deciding not to check emails or texts after a particular hour, allowing you to unwind and recharge. Or you might set a boundary around your personal space, choosing not to share specific details with everyone. These boundaries are not about building walls but placing gates where needed, ensuring that the interactions and responsibilities you engage with are your choosing and within your capacity to handle.

Identifying the areas where boundaries are needed might seem daunting, but it starts with tuning in to your feelings. Notice moments when you feel discomfort, resentment, or exhaustion—these are often signs that a boundary is being crossed.

If you feel constantly drained after interactions with a particular friend, it might be time to set a boundary around how much time you spend with them or what topics you want to discuss. Similarly, if schoolwork encroaches on your time, creating clear boundaries around study hours and relaxation time can help maintain balance.

Enforcing Boundaries

Once you've identified where boundaries are needed, the next step is learning how to assert them respectfully and effectively. Saying no is a powerful part of this process. It's about being clear and direct with your needs without being dismissive or offensive.

For example, if a friend asks you to help with a project and you don't have the time, instead of an abrupt "I can't," you might say, "I want to help, but I have my commitments now. Can we find another time or way I can assist?" This approach acknowledges the request and shows your willingness to help while standing firm on your availability.

Respect: A Two-Way Street

Respecting others' boundaries is just as important as establishing your own. It's about recognizing and honoring the limits others set, which can differ significantly from yours. This mutual respect creates a foundation of trust and understanding in relationships, which is essential for healthy interactions.

When someone tells you no, accepting their decision without argument or judgment demonstrates that you value their needs and autonomy. This reciprocal respect for boundaries strengthens relationships and sets a standard for how you expect to be treated in return.

Setting and respecting boundaries is not a one-time task but an ongoing process that evolves with your relationships and circumstances. It requires continuous attention and adjustment as you grow and learn more about yourself and others. By mastering the art of saying no and setting boundaries, you empower yourself to interact with the world on your terms, leading to a healthier, more balanced life.

As you navigate your daily interactions, remember that each boundary set is a step toward self-respect and personal freedom, providing the space and peace needed to thrive in all areas of your life.

4.3 Difficult Conversations with Parents

When the time comes to sit down and have a stern talk with your parents—whether it's about a drop in grades, a disagreement on curfews, or something as personal as your mental health—it's natural to feel a bit apprehensive. These conversations are rarely easy, but with the proper preparation, they can become productive dialogues that deepen understanding and strengthen your relationship.

Start by planning what you want to discuss. Be clear about your thoughts and feelings, and consider jotting down the key points you want to convey. This preparation ensures you stay on track and cover all the necessary topics without getting sidetracked.

Appropriate Time

Choosing the right time and setting is crucial. You want a moment when neither you nor your parents are rushed or distracted. It might be after dinner at home or during a quiet afternoon. The calm environment contributes to a more focused and open conversation. Anticipating how your parents might react can also help you prepare responses or solutions to potential concerns they might raise. For instance, if you're discussing a drop in your grades, be ready to discuss your plan to improve them, showing you're proactive and responsible.

Importance of Communication

Effective communication goes beyond just talking. It's also about how you convey your message. Techniques like active listening, which involves giving full attention to the speaker, nodding, and offering small verbal affirmations like "I understand" can make a significant difference. This approach respects the other person's feelings and viewpoints, fostering a more compassionate dialogue. Maintaining eye contact is another vital aspect of effective communication—it helps build trust and shows sincerity. Keeping an even tone is also crucial; it conveys calmness and helps prevent the conversation from escalating into an argument.

Managing Emotional Responses

Managing emotional responses from both sides is another critical aspect of navigating difficult conversations. It's natural for emotions to run high, especially when discussing sensitive issues. Before the conversation, take some time to center yourself with a few deep breaths or a short walk. This preparation can help you enter the discussion with a calm mindset, making it easier to maintain composure if the conversation gets tense. If you get overwhelmed during the talk, don't hesitate to ask for a brief pause. A few moments of silence help everyone regain composure and approach the discussion with renewed clarity.

A Third Party

Despite your best efforts, sometimes conversations with parents go differently than planned. If you find it challenging to communicate effectively, or the discussions frequently become heated or unproductive, it might be time to seek external support. This could be a school counselor, a trusted teacher, or a family friend. These individuals can offer guidance, provide mediation, and sometimes lend a sympathetic ear. They might also have additional insights or suggestions from their experiences, which can be invaluable in finding a resolution.

Navigating difficult conversations with parents is a skill that develops over time, with each discussion providing a learning opportunity. By thoroughly preparing, communicating effectively, managing emotions wisely, and knowing when to seek external support, you can turn challenging talks into constructive experiences that enhance understanding and strengthen relationships. These conversations are essential stepping stones to becoming more thoughtful, adaptable, and communicative.

4.4 Discussing Mental Health with Parents

Talking about mental health with your parents can feel overwhelming, but it's crucial for your well-being and fostering support within your family. The key to a successful conversation lies in preparation and timing. Choose a relaxed, distraction-free moment, like a quiet evening or weekend afternoon, to talk. Avoid times when anyone is rushed, stressed, or upset.

Preparing

Preparation involves thinking about what you want to communicate. Describe your feelings, how long you've felt this way, and what might be contributing to your mental state. Writing down a few main points can help keep the conversation on track and ensure you don't forget anything important.

Express Yourself Clearly

Expressing your feelings clearly and effectively is essential. Use 'I' statements to articulate your experiences and emotions. For example, instead of saying, "You don't understand me," say, "I feel like I'm not being understood when I talk about my stress." This approach helps convey your feelings without blaming the other person, reducing the likelihood of a defensive response. The goal is to share your experiences and needs, not to assign fault.

Educate and Inform If Necessary

Educating your parents about your mental health can bridge gaps in understanding and encourage more supportive responses. Parents might not always recognize mental health issues or may understand them differently due to generational, cultural, or personal biases.

Offering them resources, like articles, books, or videos, can help expand their knowledge. For instance, if you're dealing with anxiety, find a well-reviewed article that explains what anxiety is, how it affects people, and what kind of support can help. This can turn an emotional conversation into an informative discussion, opening avenues for empathy and support.

Resistance

Even with the best preparation, be ready for resistance or misunderstandings. Not everyone is comfortable talking about mental health, and some might initially respond with skepticism or dismiss your concerns.

If this happens, try to stay calm and patient. Reiterate your feelings and the facts you've shared. Sometimes, giving the other person time to process the information can make a significant difference. If misunderstandings persist, suggesting family counseling or mediation where a neutral third party can facilitate more effective communication might be helpful.

Navigating this conversation requires courage and preparation but opens the door to greater understanding and support. By choosing the right time, expressing your feelings clearly, providing educational resources, and being prepared for different responses, you can lay a foundation for ongoing support and empathy from your family. This conversation is significant in managing your mental health and building stronger, more supportive family relationships.

4.5 Dealing with Family Conflict

Navigating family conflicts can feel like finding your way through a dense forest without a map. You know you need to get to the other side, but the path needs to be clarified, and obstacles keep popping up. Understanding the dynamics of family conflicts can help you find that map, making the journey less daunting and more manageable. Disputes within the family are typical and can stem from various sources, such as misunderstandings, differences in values or beliefs, and pressures from external sources like school or work. These conflicts can escalate quickly if not managed properly, leading to strained relationships and a tense home environment.

Underlying Reasons

Understanding why they happen is one of the first steps in managing family conflicts. Often, what seems like a minor issue might be a surface expression of deeper problems. For example, a fight over a seemingly minor issue, like a forgotten chore, reflects underlying feelings of being taken for granted. Recognizing these underlying causes can help address the root of the conflict rather than just the symptoms. It's also important to understand that each family member may have different communication styles and emotional needs, affecting how conflicts arise and escalate. For instance, one person's direct approach might appear aggressive to someone who prefers a more subtle communication style.

Effective Communication

Effective communication strategies become crucial once you understand the dynamics and causes of family conflicts. Techniques such as active listening, where you focus on what the other person is saying without planning your rebuttal, help clarify misunderstandings and show that you value the other person's perspective.

Demonstrating empathy, or the ability to put yourself in someone else's shoes, can also help de-escalate conflicts by showing understanding and care for the other person's feelings. Negotiation is another crucial strategy. This involves finding a compromise that acknowledges and addresses the needs of all parties involved. For example, if the conflict is about how much time is spent on family activities, negotiating a schedule that balances family time with personal time could be a solution.

Manage Your Emotions

Managing your emotions plays a critical role in resolving conflicts. When tensions rise, it's easy to let emotions take over, leading to escalated conflicts and hurt feelings. Techniques for staying calm and composed include taking deep breaths, stepping away from the situation to cool down, or using calming phrases like, "I need a moment to think." Keeping your emotions in check helps maintain a clear head, making it easier to work through the conflict without causing additional harm.

Follow Up

After a conflict is resolved, it is important to take steps to repair and strengthen the relationship. This might involve discussing what was learned from the experience, which can help prevent similar conflicts in the future. Expressing appreciation for the other person's willingness to resolve the conflict can reinforce positive interactions and strengthen bonds. For example, saying something like, "I appreciate your willingness to work this out with me," can go a long way in healing and improving the relationship.

Addressing family conflicts effectively requires understanding their causes, utilizing effective communication techniques, managing emotional responses, and taking steps to repair relationships after the conflict.

By developing these skills, you can navigate family conflicts more effectively, leading to a more harmonious and supportive family environment. Remember, the goal isn't to avoid disputes altogether but to handle them in a way that strengthens relationships and fosters understanding among family members.

4.6 Setting Boundaries at Home

In the complex dynamics of family life, setting boundaries is like drawing a map that shows where your territory begins and ends. It's about defining what you are comfortable with, how you expect to be treated, and what you are willing to tolerate. These boundaries are essential for maintaining your well-being and healthy relationships with your family members. Understanding and respecting each other's boundaries leads to a more harmonious and supportive home environment.

Types of Boundaries

Boundaries come in various forms and serve different purposes. Emotional boundaries help you manage who has access to your feelings and how deeply you engage emotionally with others. For example, you might choose to share your feelings about a bad day at school only with those family members who respond with empathy and support rather than those who might dismiss or belittle your feelings.

Physical boundaries involve your personal space and physical touch. Setting these boundaries might mean asking family members to knock before entering your room or respecting your decision not to engage in physical greetings like hugs if you're uncomfortable with them. Time boundaries are also crucial, especially for a busy teen. These include setting aside time for homework, rest, and activities you enjoy without feeling pressured to be constantly available to others.

Share Your Boundaries

Communicating these boundaries clearly and assertively to your family is critical. Start by choosing a calm time to discuss your needs rather than in the heat of a conflict. Explain why these boundaries are important and how they contribute to your well-being. For instance, you might say, "I need some quiet time after school to decompress and focus on my homework. It helps me manage my stress and perform better academically."

When you express your boundaries this way, you're not just stating rules. You're sharing part of your self-care routine and inviting your family to support you.

Consistency

The reality is that not all boundaries are always respected. When a boundary is crossed, it's essential to address it promptly. Reaffirm your boundaries calmly and clearly. If your younger sibling barges into your room while you're studying, remind them of your need for privacy and the agreement to knock first. Be consistent in enforcing your boundaries, which helps others take your needs seriously.

If issues persist, it might be necessary to seek external support. This can be a family counselor who can provide mediation and help all family members understand the importance of respecting each other's boundaries.

Setting and communicating boundaries is an ongoing process that requires patience and persistence. It is also dynamic, as the boundaries you need might change as you grow and your family's circumstances evolve. Regularly revisiting and adjusting these boundaries ensures they continue to serve your needs and contribute to a respectful and supportive family environment.

Remember, setting boundaries isn't about creating distance but about building a framework where everyone can coexist harmoniously, ensuring individual and collective well-being.

4.7 Supporting Siblings Through Emotional Understanding

In the dynamic landscape of family life, siblings' relationships often fluctuate between being each other's closest allies and competitors. Understanding and navigating these relationships can significantly impact your family's harmony, as well as your personal and emotional development. A crucial aspect of this dynamic is learning how to build and maintain strong emotional connections with your siblings, which can lead to a more supportive and understanding family environment, essential during both good times and bad.

Building Connections

Building emotional connections with siblings often begins with spending quality time together. This doesn't necessarily mean grand gestures but finding moments for shared experiences and activities that both of you enjoy. Whether playing video games, watching a favorite TV show, or engaging in outdoor activities, these shared moments can serve as a foundation for deeper emotional bonds.

During these activities, take the opportunity to share your thoughts and feelings. Opening up about your personal experiences can encourage your siblings to do the same, fostering a deeper understanding and empathy between you. This mutual exchange of feelings and experiences strengthens your bond and builds a safe space where each of you feels valued and understood.

Recognizing Distress

Recognizing signs of emotional distress in your siblings is another critical aspect of supporting them. Changes in behavior, such as withdrawal from family activities, unexplained irritability, or a decline in academic performance, can often signal that something is troubling them.

Approach these signs with sensitivity and care. Offering a listening ear and asking open-ended questions like, "I've noticed you seem a bit down lately. Want to talk about it?" can encourage them to open up about their feelings. It's important to listen without judgment and offer support, whether simply being there to listen, providing comfort, or helping them find professional help if the situation calls for it. By being attentive and supportive, you help alleviate their immediate distress and reinforce your role as a trusted ally in their lives.

Sibling Rivalry

Navigating sibling rivalry is another common challenge. This rivalry often stems from competition for parental attention, comparisons, or conflicts over shared resources like space and belongings. Understanding the root causes of these conflicts can lead to fairer solutions and healthier interactions.

For example, if rivalry stems from competition for parental attention, discuss how this makes you feel with your parents and work together to find ways to ensure everyone feels equally valued and loved. When disputes arise, focus on finding solutions and acknowledging and respecting each sibling's needs and perspectives. Taking turns, setting shared rules, or negotiating compromises can help manage these conflicts effectively.

Modeling Healthy Practices

Finally, role-modeling healthy emotional practices play a pivotal role in positively influencing your siblings. By practicing open communication, showing empathy, and managing your emotions effectively, you set a positive example for them.

Engage in regular self-care practices and invite your siblings to join you in activities that promote well-being, such as exercise, reading, or hobbies. Demonstrating these behaviors helps you maintain your emotional health and teaches your siblings valuable skills for managing their emotions. This can foster a family environment where healthy emotional practices are the norm, benefiting everyone's mental and emotional well-being.

By building strong emotional connections, recognizing and responding to signs of distress, effectively managing sibling rivalry, and role-modeling healthy emotional behaviors, you can significantly enhance the quality of your relationships with your siblings. These efforts contribute to a supportive, understanding, and resilient family dynamic where each member feels valued and empowered. As you continue to strengthen these bonds, remember that each step you take benefits your sibling relationships and enriches your family's emotional landscape as a whole.

4.1 Navigating Social Media and Online Interactions

Welcome to the digital jungle, where likes, comments, and DMs can send your emotions on a rollercoaster ride faster than you can double-tap an Instagram post. Let's break down how to navigate this terrain without losing your cool (or your mind).

Understanding the Impact of Social Media on Emotions

- The Comparison Trap: Seeing everyone's highlight reels can make you feel like your life is boring in comparison. Remember, social media is curated—you're seeing people's best moments, not their everyday struggles.
- FOMO (Fear of Missing Out): Seeing friends hanging out without you can trigger feelings of exclusion. But remember, you can't be everywhere at once, and that's okay!
- Validation Seeking: Getting likes and comments can give you a temporary mood boost, but relying on this for self-esteem is like building a house on quicksand.
- Information Overload: Constant exposure to news (often negative) and others' opinions can be overwhelming and anxiety-inducing.
- Filter Bubble Effect: Social media algorithms can create echo chambers, limiting your exposure to diverse viewpoints and potentially reinforcing negative thought patterns.
- Cyberbullying and Online Harassment: The anonymity of the internet can bring out the worst in some people, leading to hurtful comments and behavior that can seriously impact your mental health.

4.8 Expressing Emotions Through Art and Writing

Art and writing are not just avenues for creativity but are profound tools for emotional expression and processing. When you paint a picture or write a poem about your feelings, you're doing more than just creating; you're unpacking complex emotions in a way that can be seen and understood by yourself and others.

This process can lead to significant insights about your emotional experiences, providing a form of release that can be incredibly therapeutic. Expressing yourself through art and writing allows you to externalize feelings that might be too difficult to vocalize, offering a safe space to explore and confront these emotions.

Whether it's a painting that captures your sadness or a journal entry that articulates your anxieties, each creation acts as a step toward understanding and managing your feelings more effectively.

Journaling

Getting started with creative expression doesn't require special skills or expensive materials. It's about using whatever means you feel most comfortable with to express your inner world. Keeping a journal is one of the simplest and most effective ways to begin. It can be a digital diary on your phone, a classic notebook, or whatever feels right for you.

The key is consistency. Try to write regularly about how

you're feeling or what's happening in your life, even if it's just a few sentences each day. Over time, this journal can become a valuable tool for tracking your emotional changes and growth.

Visual Art

Sketching or drawing provides another accessible entry point into artistic expression. You don't need to be an artist; it's all about putting pencil to paper and letting your emotions guide your hand. Start with abstract shapes and colors that represent your feelings. If you're angry, you might use sharp lines and dark shades. If you're happy, perhaps bright colors and fluid shapes. This is about expressing emotion, not creating a masterpiece.

Making digital art can be a fantastic way to express emotions for those who are more comfortable with digital tools. Programs and apps allow you to create artwork that can be as simple or complex as you like, using a variety of virtual brushes, tools, and colors. The undo button alleviates the fear of making 'mistakes,' encouraging freer emotional expression.

Sharing

Sharing your artistic creations can be rewarding but also daunting. It's essential to choose how and where you share your work carefully. Online platforms can be a great place to connect with others who share your interests and may provide feedback and support. However, it is crucial to select platforms known for their supportive communities and be aware of the privacy settings available. Sharing art can make you feel vulnerable, so it's essential to ensure you do so in a safe environment where your emotional expression will be met with respect and understanding.

Art Therapy

Art therapy offers a structured approach to using art for emotional and psychological healing. This form of treatment is facilitated by professionals trained to help you explore your emotions through art. Art therapy sessions can provide guidance and support, allowing you to delve deeper into your feelings in a structured environment.

For those who might not have access to professional art therapy, many online resources and books can guide you in using artistic expression therapeutically. These resources often include prompts and exercises designed to help you explore various aspects of your emotional life through creative activities.

Whether you keep your art private or share it with the world, creating can be a powerful emotional expression and healing tool. By engaging with art and writing, you're not just making something external but also building a deeper connection with your internal world, fostering resilience and a greater understanding of your emotions. As you continue exploring these expressive avenues, remember that each piece you create reflects your journey, a snapshot of your current emotional landscape.

4.9 Music as a Mood Regulator

Have you ever noticed how a particular song can lift your spirits, calm your nerves, or pump you up? Music is not just a source of entertainment but a powerful tool for emotional regulation.

The impact of music on mood is profound and multifaceted. It involves elements such as tempo, melody, and lyrics, each playing a unique role in influencing how we feel. Faster tempos can energize and motivate, while slower tempos are soothing. Melodies in significant keys are often perceived as cheerful and uplifting, whereas those in minor keys might evoke sadness or melancholy. Lyrics can resonate personally, articulating emotions that you might struggle to express yourself or providing comfort through shared experiences.

Playlists

Creating personalized music playlists is an excellent way to harness music's mood-regulating power to meet your specific emotional needs. Start by identifying different scenarios or feelings where music could be beneficial. For instance, you might want playlists to calm anxiety, boost your mood, or provide motivation during workouts.

For each scenario, choose songs that elicit the desired emotional response. When you're anxious, songs with slow tempos and gentle melodies can be incredibly soothing. Conversely, upbeat and energetic tracks can be just the ticket when needing a mood lift. Organizing these songs into dedicated playlists ensures you have them ready whenever you need them, turning your music library into a personalized emotional toolkit.

Make Music

Encouraging active participation in music-making can further enhance its therapeutic benefits. Whether singing, playing an instrument, or composing, engaging with music creatively allows for a more profound emotional expression and connection. Making music can be a cathartic experience, offering a sense of release and a way to process complex feelings.

It can also be gratifying, instilling a sense of achievement and boosting self-esteem. If you're new to music making, start with simple instruments like the ukulele or keyboard, which are relatively easy to learn. Joining a band or ensemble can also be a great way to enhance your skills while connecting with others who share your passion for music.

Lyrics Analysis

Analyzing the lyrics of your favorite songs can also provide deeper insights into your emotions and experiences. Take some time to listen to the words, looking up the lyrics to ensure you understand them correctly. Consider what the songwriter is expressing or describing. Do these themes resonate with your feelings or experiences? How do the lyrics influence your interpretation of the song?

This analysis can deepen your appreciation of the music and help you connect with your own emotions on a more profound level. It can be particularly enlightening to explore songs that evoke strong emotional responses in you, whether it's joy, sadness, nostalgia, or hope. By understanding the elements that trigger these emotions, you can become more attuned to your emotional triggers and responses in music and life.

Incorporating music into your emotional regulation practices offers a dynamic and enjoyable method to enhance your mood, cope with stress, and express your feelings. Whether through creating personalized playlists, engaging in music making, or analyzing lyrics, music provides a versatile and accessible tool for emotional exploration and expression.

As you continue to explore the role of music in your emotional landscape, remember that each note, each lyric, and each melody offers an opportunity to deepen your understanding of yourself and your emotions, harmonizing the soundscape of your life with the rhythm of your feelings.

4.10 Dance/Movement Therapy: Body Awareness as Emotional Outlet

Discovering dance/movement therapy (DMT) opens a new way to manage emotions through movement. This form of therapy is based on the idea that our minds and bodies are deeply connected. By moving with intention, we can gain profound emotional insights and relief. DMT isn't about performing perfect dance steps but using movement to connect with and express your feelings.

Embodiment: The Heart of DMT

At its core, DMT is all about "embodiment"—the idea that physical movement can lead to deeper emotional awareness and healing. This therapy encourages you to explore new ways to move and notice how these movements make you feel. For instance, big, expansive movements might make you feel joyful and free, while small, curled movements could reflect feelings of insecurity or sadness. By practicing DMT regularly, you can develop a richer understanding of your emotions, which can help you manage them better.

Simple Movement Activities

You don't need a dance background to benefit from DMT. Simple activities can be easily integrated into your daily routine. For example, try free dancing by letting your body move to music that you love without any planned choreography. You could also try guided movement meditations, where someone leads you through movements designed to release stress and increase mindfulness. Another option is expressive gesture exercises, where you use gestures to express emotions like anger, happiness, or confusion. These activities encourage spontaneity and creativity, making emotional expression through movement fun and liberating.

Connecting Body and Emotion

DMT helps you tune into the physical sensations that come up during movement. You might notice tension in your shoulders as you dance or feel your heart race during an energetic sequence. By paying attention to these sensations, you can start to connect your physical and emotional states. For instance, if you realize that you hold tension in your shoulders when you're anxious, you can incorporate shoulder rolls or stretches into your movement practice to help relieve both the physical and emotional stress.

The Benefits of Group Dance Activities

Joining group dance activities can enhance the benefits of DMT. Participating in a dance class or workshop offers structured guidance and the social aspect of moving with others. This communal experience can be very supportive, providing a sense of connection and shared experience that can be comforting during emotional distress. Being part of a group also allows you to witness and share a range of emotional expressions, which can help normalize your feelings and offer different perspectives on handling emotions through movement.

Incorporating DMT into Your Life

Adding dance/movement therapy to your life offers a dynamic way to understand and manage your emotions. It connects physical and emotional health and provides a playful, creative outlet for expression and healing. Whether you practice at home or join a group, DMT invites you to move, explore, and express in ways that can bring significant emotional relief and insight. As you continue to navigate your emotions, remember that each step is not just a move but a powerful expression of your inner experience, creating a rhythm that resonates with your true self.

In this chapter, we've explored various facets of emotional expression and communication. We've learned about assertiveness, setting boundaries, and navigating difficult conversations with family. We've discovered how creative outlets like art, writing, and music can help regulate our moods and express our feelings. We've also examined the impact of social media on our emotions and explored physical movement as an emotional outlet.

These diverse tools and techniques form a comprehensive toolkit for understanding and expressing our emotions effectively. By practicing these skills, we can build stronger relationships, maintain better mental health, and express our authentic selves more clearly. Remember, healthy emotional expression isn't just about venting feelings—it's about understanding them, communicating them clearly, and finding constructive ways to channel them.

Chapter 5
Anxiety

I magine you're on a stage, a spotlight shining down, with hundreds of gazes on you, and suddenly, your mind goes blank. That wave of cold panic that sweeps over you doesn't just happen in public speeches. It's a familiar guest during exams, performances, or even new social settings. This chapter is about understanding and managing specific emotions like anxiety, which can feel as though they're taking the steering wheel and driving you into a storm. Here, we will equip you with the tools to navigate these emotions, not by avoiding them but by understanding and managing them effectively.

5.1 Managing Anxiety: Practical Tips and Tricks

While a little anxiety is normal (hello, butterflies before a big presentation), too much can seriously impact your health.

Anxiety vs. Worry: What's the Difference?

Normal worry is usually about specific situations and doesn't interfere with your daily life.

Anxiety tends to be more persistent and intense and can impact your ability to function.

Common Signs of Anxiety

Physical:

- Racing heart
- Sweating
- Trembling or shaking
- Stomach upset
- Headaches
- Trouble sleeping

Emotional:

- Excessive worry or fear
- Feeling on edge or restless
- Irritability
- Difficulty concentrating
- Mind going blank during stressful situations

Behavioral:

- Avoiding certain situations or places
- Seeking constant reassurance
- Procrastination
- Perfectionism
- Types of Anxiety Common in Teens

General Anxiety: Worrying excessively about various aspects of life.

Social Anxiety: Fear of social situations or being judged by others.

Test Anxiety: Intense stress specifically related to exams or evaluations.

Performance Anxiety: Fear of making mistakes in situations where you're being watched or evaluated.

Anxiety-Busting Strategies

1. Face Your Fears (Gradually)

Make a list of things that make you anxious, from least to most scary.

Start with the least anxiety-provoking situation and work your way up.

This is called exposure therapy, and it helps your brain realize these situations aren't as scary as it thinks.

2. Challenge Your Thoughts

Anxiety often involves "what if" thinking. Challenge these thoughts with evidence.

Ask yourself: "What's the worst that could happen? How likely is it? What would I do if it did happen?"

3. Breathe It Out

Try the 4-7-8 breathing technique: Inhale for four counts, hold for seven and exhale for eight.

This helps activate your body's relaxation response.

4. Get Moving

Exercise is a natural anxiety-buster.

Even a short walk can help clear your head and reduce anxiety.

5. Mindfulness and Meditation

Practice being present in the moment instead of worrying about the future.

Try guided meditations or mindfulness apps like Headspace or Calm.

6. Limit Caffeine and Sugar

These can mimic or worsen anxiety symptoms.

Pay attention to how these affect your anxiety levels.

7. Create a Worry Time

Set aside a specific time each day to focus on your worries.

Outside of this time, try to postpone worrying thoughts.

8. Use Positive Self-Talk

Develop a mantra or positive phrase to use when anxiety hits.

Example: "I've got this" or "This feeling will pass."

9. Get Creative

Engage in activities that require focus and creativity.

This can help redirect your mind from anxious thoughts.

10. Seek Support

Talk to friends, family, or a counselor about your anxiety.

Remember, asking for help is a sign of strength, not weakness.

Identifying Triggers and Preparing Responses

Anxiety isn't just a fleeting worry. It can feel like a persistent shadow, coloring your thoughts and actions, often without an apparent reason. However, by identifying what triggers your anxiety, you can prepare and respond more effectively, regaining control over how you feel and react. Triggers can be as varied as an upcoming test, a family conflict, or an overwhelming schedule. They can sneak up on you, turning an ordinary day into a whirlwind of stress.

First, start by mapping out what specifically sparks your anxiety. This could be social situations, performance scenarios like exams or presentations, or even specific thoughts about your future. Keeping a journal can be incredibly helpful here. Detail situations that increase your anxiety and note how you react. Do you withdraw? Do you become irritable? Do you procrastinate? Understanding these patterns is the first step in managing them.

Once you've pinpointed your triggers, the next step is preparing your responses. This doesn't mean scripting your life but having a toolkit ready to help you cope. Preparation might involve strategies like deep-breathing exercises, mindfulness practices, or speaking with a counselor or therapist. For instance, if you know that social gatherings trigger anxiety, you might prepare by planning strategic timeouts during the event to practice breathing exercises. Or, if exams cause stress, part of your preparation could involve setting up a study schedule that breaks down the material into manageable chunks, reducing the overwhelm.

Creating these strategies isn't just about managing moments of anxiety but about building a lifestyle that helps prevent the severity of its impact. This means regular exercise, sufficient sleep, and a balanced diet, all of which are crucial to your overall mental health, as previously mentioned. It also means building supportive relationships where you can freely express your feelings and concerns without fear of judgment. These relationships can provide emotional comfort and practical advice and support when you're feeling anxious.

Lastly, educate yourself about anxiety. Understanding that

anxiety is a common and natural response can sometimes make it feel less daunting. Knowledge empowers you to demystify the experience of anxiety and to approach it with practicality rather than fear. Numerous resources—books, articles, workshops, and videos—can offer insights and techniques for managing anxiety. The more you understand it, the better equipped you are to deal with it effectively.

In managing anxiety, the goal is not to eliminate it—that's neither possible nor beneficial, as anxiety can be a motivator, pushing you to prepare and perform. Instead, the aim is to understand and manage it so that it doesn't prevent you from enjoying life or achieving your goals. By identifying triggers and preparing responses, you take the necessary steps toward regaining control over your emotional life, turning what once felt like overwhelming obstacles into manageable challenges.

5.2 Grounding Exercises for Panic Attacks

When panic strikes, it feels like you're losing control over your mind and body, and the world starts spinning uncontrollably. That's where grounding techniques come into play. These simple, powerful strategies are designed to anchor you, pulling your attention away from the panic and returning to the present moment. Grounding can be a lifesaver during a panic attack, offering a way to regain control by focusing on the here and now rather than the overwhelming sensations and thoughts of panic.

Understanding Grounding Techniques

Grounding techniques work by diverting your focus from the internal feelings of fear and anxiety to external or physical sensations, helping break the cycle of escalating panic. They essentially 'ground' you, like a grounding wire prevents unnecessary and dangerous electric charges. By consciously shifting your focus to the present moment, you can stabilize your emotional state and reduce the intensity of the panic attack. This method is not just about distraction. It's also about connecting with the present moment to calm and reassure your mind and body that you are safe.

Physical Grounding Exercises

One effective grounding method is the "5-4-3-2-1" technique, which engages all five senses to help stabilize your emotions. Here's how to do it:

- Five: Look for five things you can see around you. It could be a poster on the wall, a spot on the ceiling, or simply the way light plays on surfaces.
- Four: Feel four things you can touch around you. This could be the texture of your clothing, the calm surface of a table, the grass under your feet, or even your hair.
- Three: Listen for three sounds you can hear. It could be the distant sound of traffic, the hum of a refrigerator, or voices in another room.

- Two: Smell two things you can smell. If you're indoors, there may be a scent of a pencil or a faint smell of coffee from your morning. If you can't immediately find smells, recall your two favorite scents.
- One: Taste one thing you can taste. This could be the lingering taste of a meal, gum, or just the inside of your mouth.

This exercise forces you to focus on your current environment and draws your attention away from the source of your anxiety. It's beneficial because it's simple and can be done anywhere, anytime, without special tools or preparations.

Mental Grounding Techniques

Mental grounding techniques involve focusing on something other than your anxious thoughts. One way to do this is by reciting something from memory. It could be anything from the lyrics of your favorite song, a poem, or a speech from a movie. The key is to focus all your mental energy on recalling the words as accurately as possible. Another technique is to play a mental game with yourself, such as counting backward from one hundred by sevens or thinking of fruit for every letter of the alphabet. These activities distract your mind from panic and help restore your sense of control.

Practice Scenarios

To get comfortable with grounding techniques, it's helpful to practice them in a controlled environment before you find yourself in the middle of a panic attack. You might role-play a scenario with a friend or therapist, where you pretend to experience a panic attack and walk through the steps of grounding yourself.

Alternatively, you could set aside a few minutes daily to practice these techniques, even when you're not anxious. This will help you improve and make them more effective when you need to use them during a panic attack.

Grounding techniques are essential for managing panic attacks and providing practical tools to cope with overwhelming anxiety. By learning to focus on the present and engage your senses or your mind in simple tasks, you can regain control over your emotions and reduce the intensity of your panic. Remember, like any skill, grounding takes practice to perfect, so the more you practice these techniques in everyday situations, the more prepared you will be to use them when panic strikes.

5.3 Time Management Tips to Reduce School-Related Stress

Navigating schoolwork, extracurricular activities, and personal life can sometimes feel like a juggling act bound to go awry, but guess what? With the right time management strategies, you can handle your daily tasks more efficiently, reducing stress and enhancing your ability to focus and perform well. Let's dig into some practical ways to manage your time, prioritize tasks, and create a study routine that works for you.

Prioritization Strategies with the Eisenhower Box

When handling school tasks, it's important to recognize that not everything needs to be treated with the same urgency. Learning to prioritize effectively can significantly reduce your workload stress. A handy tool for this is the Eisenhower Box, a simple yet effective method of sorting tasks into four categories:

Urgent and Important: Tasks that need immediate attention and are crucial for your goals. For example, an upcoming two-day exam falls into this category.

Important but Not Urgent: Tasks that are important for your long-term success but don't require immediate action. For instance, joining a new club might be crucial for your personal development but isn't pressing.

Urgent but Not Important: Tasks that require immediate attention but aren't critical to your goals. These can often be delegated or postponed.

Neither Urgent nor Important: Tasks that don't significantly impact your goals and can be eliminated or minimized. These tasks are usually distractions.

Using this matrix, you can visually sort your tasks, which helps you decide what to tackle first. This method clarifies what needs immediate attention and lets you understand that not everything is a crisis, easing the pressure and allowing you to focus on what truly matters.

Creating Effective Study Plans

Developing a personalized study schedule can transform the way you approach schoolwork. Start by assessing how you currently spend your study time. Are there periods where you feel more alert and absorb information better? Use those for your most challenging subjects. Incorporate varied study methods to keep things interesting—switch between reading, making flashcards, practicing problems, or teaching the material to a friend. This variety can help maintain focus and cater to different learning styles, making study sessions more effective.

Most importantly, remember to schedule breaks. Yes, breaks are just as crucial as study time. They prevent burnout and keep your mind fresh. A good rule of thumb is the 50/10 rule: Study for fifty minutes and break for ten. During breaks, do something completely unrelated to work—stretch, grab a snack, or just daydream. This brief disengagement from studying refreshes your mind, preparing it for another round of focused learning.

Utilization of Digital Tools

In our digital age, various apps and platforms can help you organize and track school assignments, making it easier to manage your workload. By leveraging these tools, you can keep your schoolwork organized and reduce the stress of potentially overlooked assignments or missed deadlines.

Todoist

Website: www.todoist.com

Features: Task management, project tracking, deadlines, and priority levels.

Trello

Website: www.trello.com

Features: Visual task boards, card sorting, checklists, and collaboration tools.

Google Keep

Website: keep.google.com

Features: Note-taking, reminders, checklists, and syncing across devices.

Microsoft To Do

Website: to-do.microsoft.com

Features: Task lists, reminders, due dates, and integration with other Microsoft apps.

MyHomework Student Planner

Website: myhomeworkapp.com

Features: Homework tracking, class schedules, and reminders.

Evernote

Website: www.evernote.com

Features: Note-taking, task management, document storage, and collaboration tools.

Forest

Website: www.forestapp.cc

Features: Focus and productivity tool helps manage time and reduce phone distractions.

Notion

Website: www.notion.so

Features: All-in-one workspace for notes, tasks, databases, and collaboration.

Building Routine and Structure

Establishing a consistent daily routine is your secret weapon against stress. It creates a predictable environment where your mind and body can operate optimally. Start by setting specific times for study, relaxation, and sleep. Consistency in your schedule reinforces your body's natural rhythms, making you more efficient. Ensure your routine includes sufficient time for rest—adequate sleep is non-negotiable when it comes to effective learning and emotional health.

Your routine might look something like this:

- Wake up at the same time each day.

- Start with a relaxing morning ritual.
- Attend school.
- Follow a structured study time with breaks in the afternoon or early evening.
- Ensure you have downtime in the evening to unwind before bed.

Regular exercise should also be part of your routine. It boosts mood and energy levels, making it easier to tackle your academic tasks.

By implementing these time management strategies, you empower yourself to handle school-related stress more quickly and confidently. Effectively prioritizing tasks, creating a personalized study plan, utilizing digital tools for organization, and establishing a consistent daily routine are all steps that foster a more manageable and successful school experience. As you refine these strategies, you will likely perform better academically and enjoy a more balanced and fulfilling student life.

5.4 Techniques for Handling Test Anxiety

Experiencing a surge of nerves before a test is as standard as the test itself, but those nerves don't have to dictate your performance. Understanding how to prepare effectively can transform your anxiety into a powerful ally that sharpens your focus and drives you to perform at your best.

Spaced Repetition Learning

- Break down information into manageable chunks.
- Review these chunks at increasing intervals.
- Uses the psychological spacing effect for better recall.
- Enhances retention and builds confidence by knowing the material deeply.

Active Recall

- Test yourself on the material rather than just reviewing it.
- Use flashcards, teach the material to someone else, or write down everything you remember.
- Strengthens memory and understanding by forcing your brain to retrieve information.
- Reduces test anxiety because you've practiced recalling the information.

Relaxation Techniques

- Address immediate physical and emotional symptoms of test anxiety.
- Practice deep, rhythmic breathing: inhale slowly for four counts, hold for four, exhale for four.
- Increases oxygen flow to the brain, helping you think more clearly.

Visualization

- Imagine yourself calm and in control in the test room.
- Prepares you mentally to face the actual situation with confidence.

Positive Self-Talk and Affirmations

- Identify and challenge negative thoughts like "I'm not good at this" or "I'm going to fail."
- Replace them with positive affirmations: "I have prepared well for this test, and I can handle it," or "I am capable and smart."
- Repeat these affirmations daily, especially on test day.
- Shifts your mindset to reduce stress and enhance performance by reinforcing self-belief.

After each test, engage in a post-test reflection. This doesn't mean obsessing over what might have gone wrong. Instead, it's about constructively analyzing your performance to refine your strategies. Ask yourself what worked well, what didn't, and how you felt during the test. Did the relaxation techniques help? Did your study methods prepare you? This reflection can be invaluable in continuously improving your approach to tests, helping you build more effective study habits and coping strategies over time.

By employing these techniques—spaced repetition for long-term retention, active recall for enhancing memory, relaxation methods to control anxiety during the test, and positive affirmations to boost confidence—you equip yourself with a robust set of tools for tackling test anxiety.

Each component plays a crucial role in preparing you for the test and helping you manage the stress and emotions that come with it. As you continue to apply these strategies, you'll likely find that your anxiety diminishes and your confidence grows in testing situations and other areas of life.

When to Seek Professional Help

If anxiety is significantly impacting your daily life—interfering with school, relationships, or activities you enjoy—it might be time to talk to a mental health professional. They can provide additional strategies and support to help you manage your anxiety effectively.

Remember, anxiety is super common, especially during the teenage years. You're not alone, and there are lots of ways to manage it. Be patient with yourself as you learn these new skills. With practice, you can take back control from anxiety and live your best life.

In this chapter, we've explored practical strategies for managing anxiety and related emotions, particularly in academic settings. We've learned techniques for identifying triggers, grounding ourselves during panic attacks, and effectively managing time to reduce school-related stress. We've also discovered methods for tackling test anxiety through proper preparation and positive self-talk.

Remember, these skills take practice to master, but with persistence, they can significantly improve your ability to handle challenging emotions and situations. While some anxiety is normal, if it's significantly impacting your daily life, don't hesitate to seek professional help. By applying these tools and techniques, you're taking important steps towards better emotional management and overall well-being.

Chapter 6
Managing Sadness and Depression

Imagine watching your favorite series, and suddenly, the screen dims. You fiddle with the remote and adjust the settings, but the vivid colors and sharp clarity you were enjoying don't return. This can be what encountering persistent sadness or depression feels like—a lingering shadow dimming the vibrancy of everyday life. It's crucial to understand the nuances of these emotional states and distinguish between a temporary gloom and a more severe condition that might need attention. This chapter will guide you through recognizing and managing these feelings, empowering you to bring the color back into your view of the world.

6.1 Distinguishing Between Sadness and Depression

Sadness is a natural response to disappointing, hurtful, or upsetting situations. It is a universal experience and a necessary part of the spectrum of human emotions, allowing us to process and eventually come to terms with loss or disappointment. Typically, this feeling dissipates over time as you come to terms with the triggering event, and it doesn't pervasively lower your ability to function in your daily life.

Depression is different—it's like sadness amplified and extended. It is a medical condition that affects how you feel, think, and handle daily activities; it is characterized by persistent and intense feelings of sadness and despair that last for extended periods—weeks, months, or even longer—and can significantly impair your ability to function at school, work, and social situations.

Depression isn't just a bad day or a brief feeling of being down. It is a serious condition that requires attention and appropriate treatment. Identifying the symptoms of depression is crucial for seeking help and managing the condition effectively.

Symptom Identification

Both sadness and depression can cause emotional pain, but the symptoms of depression are more intense and far-reaching. Symptoms include:

- **Changes in Sleep**: Depression often causes significant disruptions in sleep patterns, whether it's insomnia (difficulty falling or staying asleep) or hypersomnia (excessive sleeping).
- **Changes in Appetite**: Some lose their appetite and skip meals, leading to weight loss, while others might eat more and experience weight gain.
- **Lack of Concentration**: Difficulty focusing, making decisions, or remembering things is common in depression.
- **Loss of Energy**: Feeling fatigued daily, even when you haven't exerted yourself.
- **Loss of Interest**: A lack of interest or pleasure in all or most activities, even those you used to enjoy.
- **Feelings of Worthlessness or Guilt**: Harsh criticism of perceived faults and mistakes.

Impact on Daily Life

The effects of depression extend beyond your emotional state, impacting your performance at school, relationships with friends and family, and your personal growth. In school, the inability to concentrate can lead to a decline in academic performance, missed assignments, and decreased participation. Socially, depression often causes withdrawal from friends and activities, leading to isolation and loneliness.

In terms of personal development, the pervasive negativity can stunt your motivation to pursue goals or engage in personal hobbies and interests, leading to a cycle of inactivity and disengagement that further fuels depressive feelings.

Encouraging Self-Assessment

Understanding and acknowledging your feelings is the first step toward managing them. Regular self-assessment can help you determine whether you're experiencing temporary sadness or something more serious. Consider keeping a mood diary where you track your emotional state daily, note patterns, and identify triggers.

This practice helps you recognize the frequency, intensity, and duration of your emotions, providing valuable insights that can indicate whether you should seek professional help.

Remember, self-assessment isn't about self-diagnosis but about building self-awareness. It's a tool to understand what you're going through better so you can seek the right support if needed.

Mood Diary

To aid in your self-assessment, here's an example of how you might structure a mood diary:

- Date/Time: Note when you make the entry.
- Current Mood: Describe your emotional state using specific terms.

- Duration: Estimate how long you've felt this way.
- Possible Triggers: Identify any events, interactions, or thoughts that might have influenced your mood.
- Impact on Activities: Record any effects on your daily activities or interactions.
- Self-Care Actions: List your actions to care for yourself during this time.

This mood diary helps track trends and encourages active engagement with your emotional health, promoting a proactive rather than reactive approach to managing your feelings.

6.2 Daily Habits for Combating Low Moods

Establishing a consistent daily routine might sound like setting your life to a metronome—monotonous and rigid—but it's more akin to composing a symphony, where each note contributes to a harmonious outcome. When you wake up, eat, and even schedule your downtime regularly, you're not just structuring your day. You're setting up a framework that supports emotional stability.

Regular routines can anchor you, providing predictability in a world that often feels anything but predictable. This sense of structure is particularly comforting when your mood is low, as it can give a sense of normalcy and control. It helps to divide your day into segments, where specific activities are designated for particular times. Not only does this help manage your time effectively, but it also ensures you balance productivity with necessary downtime, fostering a healthier mental state.

As previously mentioned, proper rest, nutrition, and physical activity are all important to your overall well-being, particularly if you're struggling with depression. You need to be at your best physically to be at your peak mentally.

Another effective tool with which you should be familiar by now is mindfulness. Incorporating mindfulness and relaxation practices into your daily routine can effectively manage stress and enhance mood. Mindfulness helps ground your thoughts in the present moment, steering your focus away from ruminating on past events or worrying about the future. These practices promote calm awareness, reducing stress and allowing you to enjoy a more peaceful state of mind. By regularly engaging in these practices, you develop a toolkit that helps in moments of acute stress and contributes to longer-term resilience against mood swings and depression.

By integrating structured routines, regular physical activity, a balanced diet, and mindfulness practices, you can create a robust framework for combating low moods and enhancing your overall emotional well-being. Each element supports the other, creating a comprehensive approach to mood management that empowers you to lead a happier, more balanced life.

6.3 When to Seek Professional Help

Deciding to seek professional help for your mental health can feel like trying to navigate a maze without a map—knowing when to take this step is crucial but often unclear. Understanding the signs that suggest the need for professional intervention is your first key. For instance, if you find yourself enveloped in persistent sadness that doesn't seem to lift, or you're withdrawing from activities and people you once enjoyed, these could be indicators that it's time to reach out for help. Other signs include:

- Experiencing overwhelming feelings of worthlessness.
- Persistent fatigue that doesn't improve with rest.
- Having thoughts of self-harm.

These symptoms suggest that your emotional state is starting to interfere significantly with your daily functioning, a clear signal that professional guidance could be beneficial.

Overcoming Stigma

The notion of seeking help for mental health issues is often clouded by stigma and misconceptions. Common fears include worries about being judged or misunderstood or concerns that acknowledging a struggle with mental health could lead to negative consequences like being treated differently by friends or family.

It's essential to recognize that seeking help is not a sign of weakness but rather a courageous step toward understanding yourself better and improving your quality of life. Mental health professionals are trained to provide support in a non-judgmental and confidential manner, aiming to offer comfort and effective strategies tailored to your individual needs.

Finding Help

Navigating the landscape of mental health services can seem daunting, but there are several pathways you can take. A good starting point is often a conversation with a trusted adult—a parent, a teacher, or another family member, who can support finding the right resources. Schools are also valuable.

Most counselors can provide initial support and guidance and refer you to a therapist or psychologist if needed. Additionally, your family doctor is a good resource for an initial assessment and can provide referrals to mental health specialists. Many regions also offer online resources and helplines that can guide you in finding local mental health services and provide immediate support if needed.

Therapy

Upon deciding to see a therapist, knowing what to expect from a therapy session can ease your mind and prepare you for the experience.

Typically, the first session is about getting to know you— your feelings, your life's context, and the issues you face. It's an opportunity for you and the therapist to decide if this therapeutic relationship is the right fit. During this session, you must be as open as you can about what you're experiencing. It might help to prepare beforehand by jotting down what you wish to discuss, including how you've been feeling, any symptoms you've noticed, and any questions about the therapy process. Therapy is a collaborative process, so being honest about your feelings and concerns is critical to effective treatment.

Overall, recognizing when you need help and taking steps to access mental health services are crucial components of taking control of your well-being. By understanding the signs, addressing common fears, and navigating the resources available, you empower yourself to seek the support you need.

Therapy or counseling can provide valuable tools and insights to manage your mental health, fostering resilience and a healthier, more joyful engagement with life. As you continue to navigate these decisions, remember that taking care of your mental health is a profound act of self-respect.

6.4 Supporting a Friend Who's Struggling with Depression

When a friend is caught in the grips of depression, the changes can be subtle at first but soon become more apparent. They might start canceling plans more often, showing less interest in activities they used to love, or their energy levels and moods might fluctuate widely.

Recognizing these signs is the first step in providing the support they desperately need. It's about noticing those changes in their behavior, mood, and engagement in daily activities. If your friend used to be the first to suggest a weekend hike and now spends most weekends curled up in bed, or if their vibrant chatter has turned into monosyllabic responses, these could be indicators they're battling something internally.

Reaching Out

Approaching a friend about their mental health requires sensitivity and care. It's vital to choose a time and place where they feel safe and comfortable, away from the chaos of daily routines. Start the conversation with openness and without judgment. Phrases like, "I've noticed you've been seeming down lately, and I'm concerned about you," can gently open the door.

Speaking with kindness and empathy is essential while acknowledging you're there to listen and support, not to diagnose or judge. Effective listening is critical—hear what they say without planning your subsequent response. Give them space to express their feelings and validate their experiences by acknowledging their pain is real and what they're going through is tough.

Support can take many forms, from practical help with daily tasks to emotional support through regular check-ins.

Knowing someone cares can make a significant difference. Gently encourage them to seek professional help if their depression is severe or prolonged. Offer to help them find a therapist or accompany them to their first appointment if they're anxious about going alone. Remember, the goal isn't to push them but to show that help is available and that they don't have to struggle alone.

Self-Care

While supporting a friend, it's crucial to maintain your mental health. It can be emotionally draining. Sometimes, you might feel out of your depth. It's okay to set boundaries for your well-being. Recognize when the emotional load is too heavy for you to handle alone, and don't hesitate to suggest additional support like counseling or to involve other friends or family members. Knowing your limits and when to seek help is not just about protecting yourself but also about being a more effective supporter of your friend.

In this chapter, we've explored the crucial differences between sadness and depression, highlighting the importance of recognizing when temporary emotions evolve into more serious conditions. We've discussed daily habits that can combat low moods, emphasizing the power of routine, self-care, and mindfulness. We've also addressed the vital topic of seeking professional help, encouraging readers to overcome stigma and take proactive steps towards mental health.

Lastly, we've provided guidance on supporting friends struggling with depression, emphasizing the importance of empathy, active listening, and maintaining one's own well-being while helping others. Remember, managing emotions—whether your own or supporting others—is a journey that requires patience, understanding, and sometimes professional guidance. By applying these insights and strategies, you're better equipped to navigate the complexities of sadness and depression, fostering resilience and emotional well-being for yourself and those around you.

Chapter 7
Overcoming Anger

Imagine you're at a concert in the middle of the crowd, and suddenly, someone shoves you from behind. Instantly, your heart races, your muscles tighten, and you can feel the heat radiating off your face. Anger surges through you.

Now, picture this: Instead of reacting impulsively, you take a deep breath, turn around, and realize it was just an accident because the person tripped. That flash of understanding transforms your anger into relief and possibly empathy. This is the power of understanding and managing anger, and it starts with recognizing what's driving your emotions.

7.1 Understanding the Roots of Your Anger

Anger is often like the tip of an iceberg—what you see on the surface is only a tiny part of a much bigger picture. Beneath that visible anger usually lies deeper emotions, such as fear, frustration, or hurt. These feelings can be uncomfortable to confront. However, acknowledging them can provide crucial insights into what's bothering you, making it easier to address the root cause than just the symptoms.

For instance, you might feel angry when a friend cancels plans at the last minute, but deeper down, you might feel hurt or undervalued. Recognizing these underlying feelings is the first step in effectively managing your response.

To better identify what's beneath your anger, try this reflective exercise. Next time you feel angry, pause and ask yourself, "What am I feeling?" Write down everything that comes to mind. Are you scared of something? Do you feel threatened? Are you disappointed in someone or even yourself? This practice can help you become more aware of your emotional triggers and prepare you to deal with them more healthily.

Recognize Triggers

Understanding what explicitly triggers your anger is crucial. These triggers can be events, behaviors, words, or even memories. Identifying them helps you anticipate and prepare for situations that might provoke anger. For example, if you know that being criticized in front of others triggers intense anger, you can prepare by developing responses or strategies to manage your feelings.

Keeping a journal can be an excellent way to track these triggers. Whenever you feel angry, jot down the context, the people involved, and what was said or done that sparked your anger. Over time, you'll see patterns that can help you predict and manage your reactions more effectively. This proactive approach helps cool down potentially heated situations and empowers you to take control of your emotional responses.

Role of Personal Values

Often, anger signals that something important to us is being threatened or violated. Our values and beliefs form the core of who we are, and when they are challenged, it's natural to react defensively. Understanding this can help you see your anger not as an enemy but as a protector of your deeply held beliefs and values. For instance, if you highly value fairness, you might get outraged in situations where you perceive an injustice.

Reflecting on what values might be linked to your anger can provide essential insights and help you navigate situations that challenge those values with greater awareness and effectiveness. It can also lead to more constructive conversations about differences in values and beliefs rather than conflicts fueled purely by emotional reactions.

Biological Factors

At its core, anger is also a biological process. When you get angry, your body's "fight or flight" response kicks in. Adrenaline is released, increasing your heart rate, blood pressure, and energy levels, preparing you to react to a perceived threat. This physiological response can be powerful and overwhelming, making it hard to think clearly and respond rationally.

The Role of Hormones and Puberty in Heightening Emotions

For teens, hormones can play a significant role in amplifying emotions, including anger and depression. During puberty, your body undergoes various hormonal changes that can impact your mood and emotional state. These hormones can intensify feelings of anger, making it harder to manage your reactions.

Puberty is a time of significant physical, emotional, and psychological change. The surge in hormones like testosterone and estrogen can lead to heightened emotional responses. These hormonal changes can cause mood swings, making it feel like your emotions are on a rollercoaster. This can result in episodes of intense anger or frustration that may seem disproportionate to the situation at hand.

Understanding this biological basis of anger can be incredibly freeing. It reminds you that experiencing anger is a normal, natural response, not something you need to judge yourself for. However, it also highlights the importance of developing strategies to calm your physiological response before it leads to actions you might regret. Techniques like deep breathing, counting to ten, or stepping away from a triggering situation can reduce the intensity of your physical response to anger, giving you space to choose how to react.

Tips For Managing Heightened Emotions, Like Anger

- **Deep Breathing**: When you feel anger rising, take slow, deep breaths. This helps calm your nervous system and reduces the physical symptoms of anger.
- **Counting to Ten**: Give yourself a moment to cool down by slowly counting to ten before reacting.
- **Physical Activity**: Engage in regular exercise to help manage stress and release pent-up energy.
- **Mindfulness and Meditation**: Practice mindfulness or meditation to increase your awareness of your emotions and develop better control over your reactions.
- **Talk It Out**: Find a trusted friend, family member, or counselor to talk about your feelings. Sometimes, just expressing what you're going through can help you feel better.
- **Healthy Outlets**: Engage in hobbies or activities that you enjoy and that help you relax.

By acknowledging the role of hormones and the changes of puberty in your emotional experiences, you can better understand and manage your reactions. This awareness, combined with the strategies we've discussed, can help you navigate your emotions more effectively, whether dealing with your own feelings or supporting a friend through theirs.

In exploring the roots of your anger, you equip yourself with the knowledge and tools to transform your experience of this powerful emotion. By understanding the more profound feelings underlying your anger, recognizing your triggers, respecting the role of your values, and managing your biological responses, you empower yourself to handle anger in healthy and constructive ways, ultimately leading to more meaningful interactions and more prosperous emotional life.

7.2 Healthy Outlets for Anger Release

Managing anger isn't just about cooling down in the moment—it's about finding sustainable, healthy ways to express this intense emotion without causing harm to yourself or others. Engaging in physical activity is one of the most effective methods for releasing the tension that builds up with anger.

Physical Outlets

Imagine channeling all that fiery energy into a sprint, feeling the wind against your face and your feet pounding on the track, each step dissipating your frustration and clearing your mind. Activities like sports distract you from the source of your anger and metabolize the stress hormones flooding your body, transforming them into a source of energy and endurance.

Similarly, less vigorous but equally physical activities like punching a pillow or even screaming into a pillow at home can provide immediate, though temporary, relief. These methods allow for a physical expression of anger, discharging the emotion safely and preventing it from escalating.

Artistic Outlets

Moving beyond physical exertion, creative expression offers a profound way to process and decode the complex feelings associated with anger.

Whether scribbling furiously in a journal, splashing bold colors across a canvas, or strumming away on a guitar, creative activities allow you to externalize what you feel in a form that can be insightful and incredibly cathartic. Writing helps by putting a narrative to your emotions, allowing you to explore the reasons behind your anger and understand the broader context of your feelings. This can be particularly enlightening by turning raw emotion into a story you can analyze, learn from, and eventually let go of. Similarly, painting or drawing provides a visual outlet for your feelings, translating anger into physical forms and colors, which can help recognize the intensity and the triggers of these feelings.

Mindfulness and Meditation

Incorporating mindfulness and relaxation techniques into your routine can also play a significant role in managing anger. As you know by now, practices such as deep breathing, meditation, or yoga do more than calm the mind. They create a state of awareness and presence that can diffuse anger.

For example, yoga combines physical postures and controlled breathing to foster physical and mental balance, resilience, flexibility, and calmness—all qualities that can help mitigate the intensity of anger.

On the other hand, meditation encourages you to observe your thoughts and emotions without judgment, teaching you to detach and let go of anger without getting engulfed by it.

These practices promote a mental state where anger can be acknowledged and examined without acting on it impulsively.

Venting

Structured venting can be a controlled and safe way to express anger. This involves articulating your feelings through spoken or written words in an environment where you feel safe and understood. Talking to a trusted friend, family member, or therapist about what's making you angry can be incredibly relieving. It offers perspective and validation of your feelings, helping you navigate the emotions rather than bottling them up.

Write It Down

Writing letters that you never send can also be particularly therapeutic. This method allows you to express all your thoughts and feelings entirely without fear of the consequences of actual confrontation. It's a way to vocalize your frustrations privately and then, quite literally, let them go—either by storing them away or destroying them. Letting go can be powerful in releasing pent-up anger and moving forward.

Be sure, if you keep them, to store these letters somewhere, they won't be found by others. You would hate for your harmless venting and release of anger to cause someone pain months or years after the incident.

You can find healthy and effective ways to release anger through physical activity, creative expression, mindfulness and relaxation techniques, and structured venting. Each approach offers a unique pathway to express and manage anger and understand and transform this challenging emotion into something constructive and potentially enriching.

7.3 Communication Skills to Express Anger Constructively

When anger flares, it's like a spark that can kindle understanding or ignite a wildfire of conflict. How you communicate in these heated moments can determine the outcome of an interaction.

It's All About "I"

One of the most effective tools at your disposal when communicating about a situation that can cause conflict or anger is using "I" statements. These expressions focus on your feelings rather than blaming others, which can help prevent the other person from becoming defensive.

For example, instead of saying, "You never listen to me," you could say, "I feel upset when I don't feel heard." This slight shift in phrasing can make a massive difference by expressing your feelings without accusing the other person, which often leads to a more receptive and empathetic response.

It's about owning and expressing your emotions without laying blame, which encourages open, blame-free communication. Practicing "I" statements can be transformative in diffusing tension and deepening your relationships through honest and respectful communication.

Actively Listen

Active listening is another crucial skill that goes hand-in-hand with using "I" statements. It involves genuinely hearing what the other person is saying and showing that you understand. This doesn't mean you have to agree with them. You are simply considering their words, which can significantly de-escalate anger.

Active listening can be practiced by summarizing what the other person has said and reflecting it to them, a technique known as reflective listening. For instance, if a friend expresses frustration about your recent unavailability, you might respond, "It sounds like you've been feeling left out because we haven't spent much time together lately."

This approach validates their feelings and opens the door to resolving the issue without blame, fostering a dialogue that invites solutions rather than conflict.

Tone and Body Language

Managing your tone and body language can also dramatically affect how your messages are received during angry exchanges. Your voice's pitch, loudness, and pace can convey more about your feelings than the words themselves. When emotions run high, it's easy for your voice to rise in pitch and volume, making the conversation feel more like a confrontation.

Keeping a calm, steady tone can help keep the interaction constructive. Similarly, body language—like maintaining eye contact, keeping your arms uncrossed, and nodding to show you are engaged—can make the conversation feel more open and less adversarial. These non-verbal cues can communicate empathy and respect, which might help cool down heated exchanges and lead to more productive dialogue.

Think It Through

Finally, pausing before responding is a powerful tool in your communication arsenal. Our first responses are often not our best in the heat of anger. By taking a moment to breathe and think before you speak, you give yourself space to consider the most constructive response.

This pause can be the difference between saying something you regret and offering a response that leads to mutual understanding. It allows you to reflect on the best use of "I" statements, gauge your tone, and deliver your message in a way that aligns with your true intentions. This moment of pause is not just about stopping yourself from saying something regrettable. It's also an opportunity to remind yourself of your communication goals and the kind of relationship you want to build or maintain.

Incorporating these skills into your daily interactions, especially when you feel angry, can change the dynamics of your conversations. It turns potential conflicts into opportunities for deeper understanding and connection. By focusing on expressing your feelings constructively, listening actively, managing your non-verbal communication, and pausing to find the correct response, you equip yourself with the tools to handle anger in a way that builds rather than burns bridges.

7.4 Resolving Conflicts Without Escalation

Conflict is a normal part of life, especially as you navigate the complexities of growing up, forming your opinions, and interacting with others who may see things differently. The issue is not the presence of conflict but how you handle it. Mastering the art of resolving conflicts without escalating the situation can save friendships, maintain peace, and build emotional intelligence.

Problem-Solving Techniques

Let's start with problem-solving techniques that emphasize collaboration over confrontation. When a disagreement arises, try brainstorming solutions together instead of focusing on who's right or wrong.

This approach involves sitting down with the other person and openly discussing each other's perspectives and needs. The goal is to find a solution that satisfies both parties or at least compromises where each person gives a little to reach a mutually acceptable resolution. For instance, brainstorming could lead to a schedule that allows equal access if you and a sibling are arguing over who gets to use the car on a weekend. This method resolves the immediate conflict and sets a precedent for constructively handling future disagreements.

Agree to Disagree

Sometimes, finding common ground might not be possible, and that's okay. Agreeing to disagree is a valuable strategy in such cases. This doesn't mean giving up or dismissing the other person's viewpoint. Instead, it's about acknowledging that it's okay to have different opinions, and these differences don't have to result in ongoing conflict.

Communicating this can be as simple as saying, "I see we're not going to agree on this, and that's all right. I respect your views and hope we can move forward without this disagreement affecting our relationship." This approach can prevent resentment and keep the situation from escalating.

Mediation

There are also times when resolving a conflict might be beyond what you can handle alone, especially if the emotions involved are intense or if the disagreement has been ongoing. Seeking mediation from a neutral third party, like a counselor or a trusted adult, can be incredibly helpful. Mediators can facilitate discussions, helping each person express their thoughts and feelings safely and constructively and guide the dialogue toward a resolution. They're trained to handle conflicts with empathy and neutrality, ensuring all voices are heard and respected.

Prevention

Lastly, preventative strategies are crucial to managing potential conflicts before they escalate. One practical approach is setting clear personal boundaries from the outset. Communicate your needs and limits to others clearly and respectfully. For example, if you need time alone to unwind after school, tell your family and ask them to respect this need.

Similarly, expressing needs early in any relationship can prevent misunderstandings and conflicts later. For instance, if you're working on a group project, clarify your expectations and understanding of each person's roles early in the process. This proactive communication can help ensure everyone is on the same page, reducing potential conflict.

By employing these strategies—collaborative problem-solving, agreeing to disagree, seeking mediation, and setting preventative boundaries—you equip yourself with a robust toolkit for dealing with conflicts to maintain relationships and promote mutual respect. These skills are vital for your personal relationships and invaluable as you move forward into more complex social, educational, and professional environments.

Moving Ahead

Navigating the terrain of anger and conflict is no small feat, but with the right tools and approaches, it's possible to manage these challenging emotions effectively. Throughout this chapter, we've explored various facets of understanding anger, from recognizing its roots and finding healthy outlets for expression to communicating constructively and resolving conflicts without escalation. The strategies discussed here are designed not just to diffuse anger or prevent conflicts but to transform these experiences into opportunities for growth and understanding.

As we close this chapter and move forward, remember that managing anger and resolving conflicts requires practice and patience. Each step you take in applying these strategies enhances your ability to handle interpersonal challenges and contributes to your overall emotional maturity and well-being. Looking ahead, we'll continue to build on these foundational skills, further exploring how to harness your emotions to foster resilience and positive relationships.

In this chapter, we've tackled the tough subjects of anger and conflict resolution. We've explored the roots of anger, including its biological basis and the role of hormones during puberty. We've discovered healthy outlets for releasing anger, from physical activities to creative expression and mindfulness practices. We've learned valuable communication skills to express anger constructively, emphasizing the power of "I" statements and active listening.

Finally, we've examined strategies for resolving conflicts without escalation, including collaborative problem-solving and mediation. Remember, managing anger and resolving conflicts are skills that improve with practice. By applying these techniques, you're not just avoiding confrontations— you're building emotional intelligence, strengthening relationships, and developing crucial life skills that will serve you well beyond your teenage years.

A Request

Have you heard the saying: "As we lose ourselves in the service of others, we discover our own lives and our own happiness." – Dieter F. Uchtdorf.

Life becomes truly fulfilling when we extend a helping hand to others. Let's join forces to make a positive impact!

Would you consider reaching out to a teenager who, just like you, is curious about The Teen's Coping Toolkit but uncertain if it's the right fit for them?

My mission is to make emotional resilience accessible to all teens.

To broaden my reach, I need your support.

Many people rely on reviews when choosing books. So, I'm appealing to you to help a teenager by writing a review.

This small act of kindness won't cost you anything and will only take a moment, but it could change someone's life. Your review could...

> ...empower one more teen to stand up to peer pressure.
> ...help one more adolescent navigate a difficult situation.
> ...boost the self-esteem of one more young person.
> ...equip one more teenager with the tools to manage their emotions.
> ...make one more dream of a happier, healthier, more confident teen a reality.

To make your impact, simply leave your review on Amazon.

If you're passionate about uplifting others, you're exactly the kind of person I appreciate. Thank you from the depths of my heart!

C.M. Krueger, PhD

Chapter 8
Self-Esteem and Self-Image

I magine you're staring at a mirror, but instead of seeing your reflection, you see a mosaic of every comment, label, expectation, and social media post ever made about you. This image may seem distorted, confusing, and even overwhelming. That's often what our self-image feels like—a complex picture influenced by external and internal factors. In this chapter, we dive into understanding self-image, how it shapes our interactions and decisions, and how you can refine this image to reflect who you are and aspire to be.

8.1 Assessing Your Self-Image: A Self-Reflection Activity

Self-image is the mental picture you have of yourself, significantly influencing your interactions, choices, and goals. It's not just about how you see your physical appearance, but also how you perceive your personality, abilities, and place in the social world. This self-perception impacts everything from the risks you're willing to take to the relationships you form. For instance, if you see yourself as unlikable, you might hesitate to engage in social interactions, missing out on potential friendships. Conversely, a positive self-image can empower you to take on challenges and embrace opportunities confidently. Understanding and occasionally reassessing your self-image is crucial because it can drift from reality over time, influenced by successes, failures, and feedback from others.

Guided Self-Reflection Exercise

To start this journey of self-discovery, I encourage you to engage in a self-reflection exercise. Find a quiet space, where you can sit comfortably without interruptions. Grab a journal or use a digital note-taking app. Here's a step-by-step guide to delve into your self-perception:

- **List Your Strengths:** Write down what you believe are your strengths. These could be skills like playing an instrument or personal traits such as empathy or resilience.
- **Acknowledge Your Weaknesses:** Objectively consider areas where you might need improvement. Remember, acknowledging weaknesses is a strength in itself.

- **Reflect on Your Achievements:** Jot down accomplishments you are proud of, no matter how big or small they seem. These can be academic, personal, or even social achievements.
- **Identify Areas for Improvement:** Think about aspects of your life you wish to improve. This could relate to skills, emotional responses, or relationships.

This exercise isn't about judging yourself but understanding and developing a more nuanced view of who you are.

Analyzing Influences on Self-Image

Our self-image doesn't form in a vacuum. It's shaped by various external influences—feedback from peers, expectations from family, and, increasingly, portrayals in the media. Reflect on the compliments you've cherished, or the criticisms that stung, and consider how these have molded your view of yourself. Family expectations can also play a significant role, setting a framework within which you might judge your successes and failures. Social media adds another layer, often presenting idealized versions of reality that can make your daily life seem inadequate by comparison. Recognizing these influences can help you differentiate between an imposed image and who you are.

Developing a Realistic Self-View

Balancing your self-perception involves recognizing and embracing both your strengths and weaknesses. It requires filtering out unrealistic standards set by external influences and focusing on personal growth. Here's a practical approach:

- **Set Personal Standards:** Define success on your terms. What matters to you the most? Is it kindness, integrity, perseverance? Let these values guide your self-assessment.
- **Embrace Imperfections:** Understand that imperfections are part of being human. They do not define your worth but are areas for personal growth.
- **Seek Feedback:** Sometimes, we are our harshest critics or greatest admirers. Obtain feedback from trusted friends or mentors to help balance your self-view.
- **Reflect Regularly:** Make self-reflection a regular practice. As you grow and change, so will your strengths, weaknesses, and achievements. Regular reflection helps keep your self-image aligned with your current reality.

This continuous process of self-reflection and assessment fosters a healthier, more accurate self-image that reflects your true self, free from the distortions of external pressures and unrealistic expectations. This authentic self-view enhances your self-esteem and empowers you to live a more fulfilled and purposeful life.

8.2 Overcoming Negative Self-Talk

Have you ever found yourself caught in a loop of self-criticism that seems to pull you down no matter what you achieve? It's like having an internal critic constantly highlighting your flaws and dismissing your successes. This is negative self-talk, and it's more common than you might think. Recognizing and transforming this internal dialogue is crucial because it significantly shapes how you view yourself and influences your behavior and emotions. Let's start by identifying the typical negative self-talk patterns and then explore strategies to rewrite these narratives into more empowering ones.

Patterns

Negative self-talk often manifests in patterns like all-or-nothing thinking, where you see things in black-or-white terms. For example, if you didn't ace a test, you might think, "I'm terrible at this subject," ignoring previous successes. Overgeneralization is another pattern, where you take one instance and generalize it to an overall pattern, thinking, "I always mess up" because of one mistake. Lastly, self-blame involves attributing every setback or problem directly to oneself, ignoring external factors or bad luck. These thought patterns can be deeply ingrained, but awareness is the first step toward change.

Cognitive Behavioral Techniques (CBTs)

Cognitive-behavioral techniques provide powerful tools to counter destructive thoughts. One effective method is to challenge these thoughts by asking yourself evidence-based questions. For example, if you think, "I never do anything right," ask yourself, "Is that really true? Can I think of times when I've succeeded?" This approach helps dismantle the absoluteness of negative thoughts and introduces a more balanced perspective.

Another technique is reframing, which involves shifting your perspective to view a situation in a more positive or realistic light. Instead of thinking, "I failed this test; I'm not smart enough," you might reframe it to, "This test was difficult, but I can learn from my mistakes and improve." This way, you transform a negative thought into an opportunity for growth and learning.

Role-Playing

Role-playing scenarios are also an excellent way to practice responding to negative self-talk. Imagine a situation where you typically experience negative thoughts and role-play a conversation with yourself, substituting negative self-talk with positive reframing or factual challenges. You can do this exercise with a friend or mentor, or even record yourself to play back and analyze. This not only helps solidify the cognitive techniques but also makes you more aware of the frequency and triggers of your negative thoughts.

Positive Affirmations

Building a habit of positive affirmations can further help

shift your internal dialogue from negative to positive. Start by identifying qualities or achievements you feel proud of and creating positive statements about them, like "I am a dedicated student" or "I am kind to my friends." Repeat these affirmations daily, ideally in front of a mirror. Over time, these affirmations can become a natural part of your thought process, gradually replacing the negative commentary.

By actively identifying harmful thought patterns, challenging them, practicing through role-playing, and reinforcing positive affirmations, you can significantly alter the landscape of your internal dialogue. This transformation boosts your self-esteem and empowers you to approach life's challenges with a more positive and balanced outlook. The goal isn't to never have negative thoughts but to not let them control or define you. As you work through these techniques, you'll find that you're speaking kindlier to yourself and feeling genuinely better about who you are and what you can accomplish.

8.3 The Impact of Social Media on Self-Esteem

We've previously discussed social media, but it bears a deeper dive. Scrolling through your social media feeds, it's easy to get swept up in images of perfect lives. Everyone seems to be on an exotic vacation, wearing the latest fashion, or flaunting achievements. It's as though you're constantly bombarded with highlights from others' lives, which can make your experiences feel less exciting or valuable. This constant exposure to idealized-life versions can seriously skew your self-image and self-esteem, making you feel like you're not measuring up. The trick isn't to avoid social media but to understand and navigate it in a way that preserves your self-esteem.

Critical Consumption Skills

Let's talk about how you can develop critical media consumption skills. It's crucial to remember that what you see on social media is often a curated representation of reality. Most people only share their best moments, carefully edited and filtered to project an image of perfection. Start by asking yourself whether your viewing is an everyday reality or a highlight reel. When you see a post that makes you feel inadequate, remind yourself that it's likely not the complete picture. There's a behind-the-scenes to every perfect post, and it often includes just as many ups and downs as your life does. To practice this, try an exercise where you compare two sets of images: Professional photos versus candid shots from various social media accounts. This can help illustrate how lighting, angles, and editing alter appearances and scenarios, emphasizing the constructed nature of social media content.

Healthy Boundaries

Setting healthy boundaries with social media is another crucial strategy. It's easy to fall into the habit of checking your phone every few minutes, but too much exposure can lead to increased feelings of inadequacy and anxiety.

Consider setting specific times of the day for checking social media, like twenty minutes in the morning and evening. If you can't easily maintain these goals, use app-limiting features on your phone or install apps that track and control your usage to help enforce these boundaries. Moreover, make it a rule not to check social media during meals or right before bed, as these are times when the adverse effects of social media can be particularly potent, disrupting both your eating patterns and sleep.

Create Your Own

Encouraging content creation rather than passive consumption can also transform your social media experience. You contribute to a more authentic online environment when you actively create and share content that reflects your real life and values. This could be as simple as sharing photos from your daily life that aren't perfectly posed or edited or posting about a cause important to you. You could start a blog or vlog discussing real issues that matter to you, like mental health, school stress, or hobbies. Creating content gives you control over your online presence and helps you connect with others who share your interests and values, fostering a supportive and engaging social media environment. It also gives you a look "behind the curtain," when you're editing and creating content. You'll soon realize just how much work goes into making a social media life seem perfect and be less influenced by the illusion.

By understanding social media's curated nature, setting boundaries to manage your consumption, and engaging in authentic content creation, you can protect and even enhance your self-esteem in the digital age. Remember, social media is a tool, and like any tool, its impact depends on how you use it. Use it wisely, and you can transform it from a source of stress into a platform for expression and connection.

8.4 Building Confidence through Achievable Goals

Be SMART

Setting goals is much like plotting a route with GPS before a road trip. It provides direction and markers that help gauge your progress. Understanding how to set practical goals is crucial for teens, especially those navigating the complex landscapes of personal and academic life. This isn't just about achieving what you set out to do. It's about building confidence and a sense of agency. The SMART criteria— Specific, Measurable, Achievable, Relevant, and Time-bound—offer a framework to set goals that aren't just wishes but achievable targets.

Be Specific

Specific goals clear the fog, showing precisely what you aim to achieve. For instance, rather than saying, "I want to get better at math," a specific goal would be, "I want to improve my math grade from a B to an A by the end of the semester." This clarity points you in the right direction and simplifies the process of achieving the goal because you know precisely what you're aiming for—measurable goals then let you track your progress.

Be Measurable

Measurable goals let you track your progress. In the math goal example, the grades on your tests and assignments provide clear milestones to measure how close you are to achieving an A.

Be Achievable

Achievability is about setting challenging yet within-reach goals, considering your current abilities and constraints. It's important to set goals that push you but are still attainable.

Be Relevant

Relevance ensures that your goals align with your larger aspirations and values, which increases your motivation to achieve them. Make sure your goals matter to you and fit into your broader plans.

Be Time-Bound

Time-bound goals have a deadline, creating a sense of urgency and helping prioritize tasks. For example, aiming to improve your math grade by the end of the semester gives you a clear timeframe to work within, helping you stay focused and on track.

Small Wins Strategy

The strategy of setting small, interim goals, or what is often called the 'small wins strategy,' is particularly effective in building momentum. Each small goal achieved is a building block toward a larger objective, and each success boosts your confidence. For example, if your overall goal is to write a novel, setting a small goal to write a chapter a month breaks down the daunting task into manageable pieces. Each chapter completed is a win, keeping your motivation high and giving you tangible evidence of your capabilities.

Track Your Progress

Keeping a journal or using an app to track your progress can significantly enhance this process. Documenting your journey keeps you accountable and provides a visual representation of your progress. Apps like Trello or Asana can help manage your goals and to-do lists, making the process less overwhelming and more structured. You might set up a board with tasks categorized under 'To Do,' 'Doing,' and 'Done.' Moving tasks to the 'Done' column can be incredibly satisfying, and a visual reminder of your accomplishments.

Celebrate Achievements

Celebrating achievements, no matter how small, is crucial. It reinforces the belief that your efforts are worthwhile and you can achieve your goals. This could be as simple as treating yourself to a movie after completing a project or spending time with friends after taking a test. These celebrations offer a well-deserved break and prepare you for the next challenge, reinforcing a positive loop of setting and achieving goals.

Through the SMART framework, the strategy of small wins, tracking progress, and celebrating achievements, goal setting becomes a dynamic tool for personal and academic success and building self-esteem and confidence. Each goal achieved is a step toward external success and internal growth, crafting a self-image rooted in real achievements and capabilities. As you continue to set and achieve goals, remember the process is just as important as the outcome, shaping you into a proactive, resilient individual ready for whatever challenges.

8.5 Turning Jealousy into a Growth Opportunity

At some point, you've probably scrolled through social media or watched a classmate receive an award and felt jealous. It's that uncomfortable sense where you find yourself wishing you had what others do, whether it's their looks, achievements, or the seemingly perfect life they portray. Understanding that jealousy often stems from our insecurities, fears, or unmet needs is the first step in transforming this feeling from a source of negativity into a catalyst for personal growth and self-improvement.

When you experience jealousy, it's usually a signal that something within you needs attention. Maybe it's an insecurity about your academic abilities, or anxiety about your social standing. By recognizing jealousy as a signpost, you can begin a journey of self-exploration to uncover these underlying issues. Start by asking yourself what specifically about the situation makes you jealous. Is it about the other person's success, or your fear of not being good enough? Understanding the root of your feelings allows you to address these deeper issues directly rather than letting jealousy control your emotions and actions.

Practicing Gratitude

One effective way to counter feelings of jealousy is by practicing gratitude. This involves shifting your focus from what you lack to appreciating what you have. Begin by making a daily list of things for which you're grateful. These don't have to be extensive or impressive. They can be as simple as a good meal, a supportive friend, or even a sunny day. The practice of gratitude brings into perspective how much you already have, and often reveals that the disparity between you and those you envy isn't as vast as it seems. Over time, this practice can significantly alter your emotional response to situations that typically evoke jealousy, fostering a sense of contentment and reducing the intensity of jealous feelings.

Change Your View

Another transformative approach is to view others' successes as opportunities for learning rather than threats to your self-worth. When someone excels in an area that you're struggling with, instead of stewing in jealousy, consider reaching out to them for advice or insights. This helps you improve in areas you feel deficient and turns potential envy into a productive learning experience. By adopting a mindset that views success as a shared or communal asset rather than a zero-sum game, you can transform jealousy into motivation, driving your personal growth and achievement.

Use It as Fuel

Additionally, use feelings of jealousy as motivators to set personal goals. If seeing someone excel in a sport makes you jealous, set a goal to improve your athletic skills. The key here is to ensure these goals are realistic and within your reach. This is where the SMART criteria—Specific, Measurable, Achievable, Relevant, and Time-bound— become useful. By setting clear, well-defined goals, you work toward overcoming your insecurities and redirecting the energy from your feelings of jealousy into constructive channels.

In essence, envy doesn't have to be a destructive force. By understanding its roots, practicing gratitude, learning from others, and setting personal goals, you can turn envy into a powerful tool for personal development. This approach alleviates feelings of jealousy, enhances self-esteem, and accelerates growth, turning potential negatives into positives.

In this chapter, we explored the nature of self-esteem and self-image, emphasizing how external influences like feedback from peers, family expectations, and social media can shape our self-perception. Through self-reflection activities, we encouraged developing a realistic and balanced view of oneself, highlighting the importance of recognizing both strengths and weaknesses. We also examined how negative self-talk can undermine self-esteem and introduced cognitive-behavioral techniques to challenge and reframe these thoughts. Additionally, we discussed the impact of social media, the benefits of setting SMART goals, and strategies to manage low moods and transform jealousy into a growth opportunity. By understanding these concepts and applying the suggested strategies, you can foster a healthier self-image and build resilience, confidence, and a positive mindset.

Chapter 9
Self-Care and Emotional Wellbeing

M aintaining your physical, mental, and emotional health is crucial, especially during the fast-paced and often challenging teenage years. Self-care is more than just occasional indulgence. It's a vital routine that ensures you can handle life's demands without burning out. This chapter explores the core of self-care, highlighting why it's essential to integrate it into your daily life. By taking care of your body, mind, and emotions, you set yourself up for success, resilience, and overall wellbeing..

9.1 The Essentials of a Teen Self-Care Routine

Defining Self-Care

Self-care often conjures images of bubble baths and spa days, but for teens like you, it encompasses much more. It's about crafting a lifestyle that balances the many aspects of wellness—physical, mental, and emotional—to sustain your health,happiness, and performance, whether at school, in sports, or in social settings. At its core, self-care means taking proactive steps to care for yourself to prevent burnout, reduce stress, and maintain your energy levels. It's about listening to your body and mind, recognizing your needs, and meeting them respectfully and kindly.

Components of a Balanced Self-Care Routine

A well-rounded self-care routine for teens should include several key components:

- **Physical Activity:** This isn't just about avoiding sedentary behavior. Regular physical activity boosts endorphins, the body's natural mood lifters. It can be anything team sports, dance classes, and other group pursuits, or simple daily stretching and walking. The goal is to move your body and enjoy it.
- **Mental Breaks:** Your brain needs rest, just as your body does. Mental breaks can involve short periods throughout the day where you step away from homework, social media, and other stressors. This might mean doing a puzzle, meditating, or sitting quietly—activities that help clear and reset your mind.
- **Social Interaction:** Spending time with friends and family who uplift and understand you is

crucial. These interactions should be nurturing and provide connection and support, helping you feel less isolated with your challenges.

- **Time for Hobbies and Interests:** Engaging in hobbies you love improves your mood and can take your mind off stressors. Whether art, music, reading, or coding, these activities provide a creative outlet and a break from routine pressures.

Tailoring Self-Care to Individual Needs

No two people are the same, and personalized self-care is most effective. You might find peace in painting, while someone else might find it through playing basketball. Listen to what your body and mind tell you. Do you feel more energized after social interactions, or do you require solitude to recharge? Adjust your self-care practices to these cues. Start small. Consider integrating a ten-minute walk into your daily routine, or setting aside time each evening to unwind with a book. The key is consistency and ensuring these activities are things you look forward to rather than see as chores.

Regular Review and Adjustment

As your life changes—and it will—your self-care needs will too. Regularly reviewing and adjusting your self-care routine is crucial. What worked during the summer might not work during a busy school semester. Perhaps you've developed new interests that you want to incorporate into your routine, or maybe you've outgrown others. This adjustment process is a normal and healthy part of maintaining an effective self-care routine. It ensures that your practices grow and evolve with you, continuing to meet your needs effectively.

Reflective Journaling Exercise

Consider starting a self-care journal to help you integrate these insights into your life. Each day, briefly record what activities you did for self-care, how they made you feel, and any thoughts on what you might want to try differently. This habit reinforces your commitment to self-care and provides valuable feedback on what's working and what's not, helping you tailor a routine that genuinely supports your well-being.

Self-care for teens isn't about escaping life but making sure you're showing up as your best self for school, relationships, and personal growth. By understanding and implementing a balanced self-care routine, you equip yourself with the tools to maintain your health and well-being amidst the pressures of the teenage years.

9.2 Sleep and Emotional Health: Making the Connection

Sleep, often relegated to merely a necessity for physical rest, is pivotal in your emotional and psychological well-being. Think of sleep as the nightly reset button for your brain. It's when your mind processes the day's experiences, regulates emotions, and consolidates memories. When you skimp on sleep, it's not just your energy levels that take a hit. Your mood, cognitive abilities, and overall mental health can suffer too. Consistent lack of sleep can make you more susceptible to stress, impede your problem-solving skills, and heighten emotional reactivity. This connection between sleep and emotional regulation is why ensuring quality sleep is crucial.

Disruptions

Disruptions to healthy sleep patterns are common among teens, often due to lifestyle choices and environmental factors. High caffeine intake incredibly late in the day can interfere with your ability to fall asleep and diminish sleep quality. Similarly, excessive screen time before bed, whether homework on a computer, or scrolling through social media on your phone, exposes you to blue light, which disrupts the natural production of melatonin, the hormone that signals your brain it's time to sleep. Moreover, irregular sleep schedules, a frequent result of juggling schoolwork, extracurricular activities, and social life, can confuse your body's internal clock and lead to sleep problems like insomnia.

Consistent Routines

To combat these disruptions and improve your sleep hygiene, establish a consistent bedtime routine that signals to your body it's time to wind down. This routine could include activities that promote relaxation, such as reading a book (not an e-book on a device), listening to soothing music, or practicing gentle yoga stretches. Aim to go to bed and wake up at the same time every day, even on weekends, to regulate your body's clock. Also, make your sleeping environment conducive to rest by keeping your bedroom cool, quiet, and dark. Use blackout curtains, eye masks, or white noise machines, if needed.

Relaxation Techniques

If you struggle with sleep despite these measures, it might be time to explore relaxation techniques to help quiet your mind and prepare your body for sleep. Techniques such as deep breathing exercises, progressive muscle relaxation, or guided imagery can be very effective. For instance, you could practice the 4-7-8 breathing technique previously mentioned: Breathe in for four seconds, hold for seven seconds, and exhale for eight seconds. This method helps reduce anxiety and induce sleepiness. If sleep difficulties persist, you must consult a healthcare provider or a sleep specialist, who can offer further guidance and, if necessary, evaluate you for sleep disorders.

Maintaining healthy sleep is not just about avoiding tiredness. It's about nurturing your mental health, enhancing your emotional resilience, and ensuring you have the energy to enjoy life and face its challenges. You equip yourself with an essential emotional and psychological well-being tool by prioritizing sleep and taking proactive steps to improve sleep quality. Remember, every good day starts the night before, so give your sleep the attention it deserves and watch how it positively transforms your mood and mental clarity.

9.3 Nutrition's Role in Mood Regulation

You are what you eat—not just physically, but emotionally too. Have you ever noticed how a sugar rush is followed by a crashing low, or how a balanced meal can keep you steady and focused? That's because the food you consume is crucial in regulating your mood, impacting everything from your energy levels to your feelings. Understanding the connection between food and mood starts with the science of neurotransmitters, the brain chemicals that communicate information throughout your brain and body. Dopamine and serotonin, for example, are neurotransmitters that heavily influence your mood and are directly affected by what you eat.

Fatty Acids, Vitamins, and Minerals

The brain requires a constant supply of nutrients from our diet to function optimally. Omega-3 fatty acids, for example, are powerful mood enhancers found in fish like salmon and sardines, as well as walnuts. They play a crucial role in rebuilding brain cells and thus help enhance neurotransmitters' function. This makes them vital not just for mental clarity but also for emotional stability.

Similarly, B vitamins in whole grains, lean meat, and fruits facilitate nerve communication and are essential for energy production, impacting stress levels and mood swings. Vitamin D, often absorbed through sunlight exposure but also available in egg yolks and fortified foods, has been linked to lowering rates of depression. Magnesium, a mineral found in leafy greens, nuts, and seeds, is known for its ability to soothe the nervous system, helping you to manage stress and sleep better.

Incorporating these nutrients into your diet isn't just about eating salads all day. It's about making intelligent, tasty choices that fuel your body and stabilize your mood. Start with simple swaps: Replace refined grains like white bread with whole grain alternatives such as quinoa or whole wheat. These contain more B vitamins and fiber, which help to regulate blood sugar levels, thus maintaining stable energy levels throughout the day. Snacking smart can also make a huge difference. Grab a handful of almonds or a banana instead of reaching for candy or chips when you're feeling down. These healthier options provide magnesium and potassium, which help enhance your mood and energy without the crash that comes from sugary snacks.

Mindful Eating

Another critical aspect of nutrition is mindful eating, which involves focusing on the experience and tastes of food rather than multitasking while you eat. Mindful eating encourages you to slow down and listen to your body's hunger cues, helping you enjoy your food more and recognize when you're full, which prevents overeating. This practice helps maintain a healthy weight and aligns you more closely with your body's needs, reducing the likelihood of mood swings associated with overeating or consuming too much junk food. To practice mindful eating, try this: At your next meal, focus on chewing slowly and appreciating the flavors and textures of your food. Turn off the TV and put away your phone. This not only improves digestion but also enhances your dietary satisfaction, which positively impacts your mood.

The relationship between what you eat and how you feel is complex and powerful. By choosing foods rich in mood-enhancing nutrients and practicing mindful eating, you can foster better physical health and a more positive and stable emotional state. Remember, each meal is an opportunity to feed your body and mood, so make choices that nourish and delight you.

In this chapter, we discussed the essential aspects of self-care and emotional well-being, emphasizing the importance of maintaining physical, mental, and emotional health. We explored how self-care goes beyond occasional indulgences, becoming a crucial routine that helps manage life's demands and prevents burnout. We covered the fundamentals of a balanced self-care routine, highlighting physical activity, mental breaks, social interactions, and personal hobbies tailored to individual needs. We also discussed how to regularly review and adjust these practices as life changes, ensuring they remain effective.

Chapter 10
The Role of Relationships in Coping

Picture yourself in the middle of a vast network, a web of threads, each connecting you to another person in your life. Some of these threads are thick and vibrant, signifying relationships that enrich your life and bolster your spirits. Others might be frayed or darkened, representing connections that may be draining or challenging. This network significantly influences your emotional landscape, impacting how you navigate joys and challenges. In this chapter, we delve into the profound role relationships play in your ability to cope with life's ups and downs, focusing on how you can cultivate a circle of relationships that genuinely supports your well-being.

10.1 Choosing Your Circle: Friendships That Foster Well-being

Friendships are not just about having fun and hanging out. They are vital sources of support, advice, and encouragement. However, not all friendships offer the same level of positivity or support. To identify genuinely supportive friends, look for qualities like trust, respect, and mutual encouragement. Trustworthy friends are those who keep your confidence and stick by your side through various challenges.

Respectful friends acknowledge your boundaries and accept your choices without judgment. Those who encourage you not only cheer on your successes but also motivate you when you're down, helping you see your potential even when you might not see it yourself. Recognizing these qualities in your peers can guide you to foster more profound, supportive relationships that enhance your ability to cope with life's stresses.

The Impact of Friendships on Mental Health

The support you receive from your friends can be a powerful buffer against mental health challenges. Studies have shown that supportive solid networks reduce loneliness, decrease anxiety, and boost overall well-being. Friends can provide a sense of belonging, which is a crucial element in maintaining emotional health. They also offer a sounding board for expressing your thoughts and feelings, which is vital to processing emotions. Moreover, friendships can help build your self-esteem. When you feel valued and accepted by your peers, you are more likely to view yourself positively. Cultivating friendships that provide emotional support and genuine companionship can be one of the most effective ways to enhance your resilience and emotional stability.

Navigating Toxic Relationships

Not all relationships contribute positively to your life. Some can be downright toxic, draining your energy and negatively impacting your mental health. Recognizing these harmful relationships is crucial. Signs of a toxic relationship may include a friend who consistently undermines your confidence, dismisses your feelings, or manipulates you. Managing such relationships often involves setting firm boundaries or, in some cases, distancing yourself from the individual. It's important to remember that ending a toxic relationship isn't a failure—it's a step toward respecting and caring for yourself.

Cultivating New Friendships

Building new friendships can be a refreshing way to expand your support network. Engaging in activities that align with your interests—such as joining clubs, volunteering, or participating in community events—can connect you with like-minded individuals. When you meet potential friends, be open and inviting but also mindful of the qualities that make up supportive friendships. It's okay to take your time to get to know new people because real connections are often built gradually. Remember, cultivating meaningful friendships can enrich your life and significantly bolster your ability to cope with your challenges.

Navigating the ups and downs of friendships and relationships can be tricky, but knowing the key qualities that make for healthy, supportive connections can really change the game. By choosing to build positive relationships and steering clear of toxic ones, you set yourself up with a strong support network that boosts your emotional and mental well-being. This proactive approach not only helps you feel good now but also builds flexibility to handle whatever challenges come your way in the future.

10.2 Handling Peer Pressure and Bullying

Imagine walking down the school hallway, caught between the urge to fit in and the desire to stay true to who you are. This tug-of-war is often the essence of peer pressure—a dynamic every teen encounters. Peer pressure isn't just about the overt offers to skip class or try something risky. It can be subtle, like a nudge to laugh at a joke you don't find funny, or to change your style to blend in with the crowd. Understanding these forces can help you navigate them without losing sight of your values.

Forms of Peer Pressure

Peer pressure morphs in various forms, sometimes appearing harmless or even supportive. For instance, it feels positive when a group of friends excites you about joining a club or trying out for a sport, but when the same group pushes you toward actions that clash with your values, that pressure can become a source of conflict. The key to handling this is recognizing when you're being swayed against your will. Start by checking in with your feelings. Are you comfortable with the decision, or are you just trying to avoid feeling left out? This reflection helps distinguish between genuinely wanting to participate and feeling compelled to conform.

Resisting Peer Pressure When resisting negative peer pressure, your self-assurance is your shield. By fostering a strong sense of self rooted in a clear understanding of your values and beliefs, you can stand firm against attempts to sway you. This doesn't mean you need to confront every peer or situation that challenges your stance. Sometimes, simply saying, "No, that's not for me," and walking away is powerful. Surrounding yourself with friends who respect your choices and encourage you to be your best self can also create a supportive buffer against negative influences.

Dealing With Bullies

Bullying is a severe form of negative peer influence that can deeply impact your mental and emotional health. It can take many forms, from hurtful words and exclusion to online harassment. Recognizing the signs of bullying is the first step in addressing it.

Recognize the Signs of Bullying:

- **Overt Actions**: Physical pushes, shoves, or other aggressive behaviors.

- **Covert Actions**: Whispers, rumors, or social exclusion.
- **Online Harassment**: Mean comments, embarrassing photos, or messages intended to belittle.

If you experience these behaviors, remember the problem lies with the bully, not you.

Strategies for Responding to Bullying:

- **Document Incidents**: Keep a record of bullying incidents. Write them down or capture screenshots of online harassment. This documentation can be crucial if you decide to report the behavior.
- **Report to a Trusted Adult**: Talk to a teacher, counselor, or parent about what you're experiencing. Reporting isn't about tattling. It's about seeking support and ensuring your safety. Schools have protocols for handling bullying, and adults can help facilitate these processes.
- **Engage in Confidence-Boosting Activities**: Join clubs, sports, or groups that interest you. Being part of supportive peer networks can boost your confidence and provide a buffer against bullying.
- **Build a Support Network**: Surround yourself with friends who respect and uplift you. A strong

support network can offer emotional reinforcement and help you feel less isolated.

By recognizing the signs of bullying and using these strategies, you can effectively address and overcome the challenges it brings. Remember, seeking help and building a supportive environment are key steps in maintaining your mental and emotional well-being.

Building Self-Esteem to Resist Peer Influence

Building resilience against peer influence starts with nurturing your self-esteem. This doesn't happen overnight but through consistent practices that affirm your worth. Here are some practical ways to boost your self-esteem:

- **Engage in Activities You Enjoy:** Do things that make you feel competent and valued, whether it's a sport, hobby, or creative pursuit. These activities can help you recognize your strengths and build confidence.
- **Set Personal Goals:** Set small, achievable goals for yourself and celebrate when you reach them. These successes, no matter how minor, can fortify your self-worth and help you feel accomplished.
- **Practice Self-Compassion:** Treat yourself with kindness, especially during tough times. Understand that it's okay to feel upset or to make mistakes. Being gentle with yourself builds a solid

foundation of self-esteem that can withstand peer pressure and bullying.

- **Daily Affirmations:** Start your day with positive affirmations. Remind yourself of your strengths and qualities. This can set a positive tone for your day and reinforce your self-worth.

- **Surround Yourself with Supportive People:** Spend time with friends and family who appreciate and support you. A positive social circle can enhance your self-esteem and provide a buffer against negative influences.

- **Reflect on Your Achievements:** Take time to reflect on what you've accomplished and be proud of your efforts. Keeping a journal can help you track your progress and see how far you've come.

- **Take Care of Your Physical Health:** Exercise regularly, eat well, and get enough sleep. Physical health is closely linked to mental well-being, and taking care of your body can improve your overall self-esteem.

By incorporating these practices into your daily life, you can build a strong sense of self-worth and resilience, making you less susceptible to peer pressure and bullying. Remember, self-esteem is an ongoing journey, but each step you take helps strengthen your inner confidence.

Navigating the complexities of peer interactions and bullying requires courage, self-awareness, and a support network. By understanding the dynamics of these challenges and equipping yourself with strategies to face them, you empower yourself to maintain your integrity and emotional well-being in the face of adversity. Every step to stand up for yourself, set boundaries, and seek support is a step toward building a more resilient and authentic you.

10.3 Setting Boundaries in Personal and Digital Spaces

Imagine your life as a series of rooms, where each room represents a different aspect: One for family, another for friends, a third for school, and yet another for your online presence. Each room has doors and windows, some of which you might want to keep open, others you might prefer to close or lock at times. This is the essence of setting boundaries—choosing where, when, and to whom you open these doors. It's a crucial skill for managing how you interact with others and let others affect you, ensuring your personal space and energy are respected and preserved.

Importance of Boundaries for Mental Health

Boundaries are essential for maintaining a healthy psyche and emotional well-being. They help you define what is acceptable and what is not, preventing others from encroaching on your emotional space. Without clear boundaries, it's easy to feel overwhelmed, taken advantage of, or exhausted, as you might constantly find yourself catering to others' needs or demands at your own expense. By setting boundaries, you protect your mental health and foster relationships based on mutual respect and understanding. These boundaries encourage supportive and empowering interactions rather than draining or demeaning.

Identifying Personal Boundaries

Identifying your boundaries starts with understanding your values, needs, and comfort levels. Consider what aspects of your life you are willing to share, and which parts you prefer to keep private. For example, you might be comfortable discussing your hobbies but not your romantic relationships. You may need a certain amount of time each day to recharge, or there are specific topics you find too personal or painful to discuss. Reflect on recent situations where you felt discomfort or irritation—it's often a sign that a boundary has been crossed. Recognizing these feelings can help you pinpoint which boundaries are important to you.

Communicating Boundaries Effectively

Once you know your boundaries, the next step is communicating them clearly and assertively to others. This might seem daunting, especially if you're worried about how others might react, but setting boundaries is a sign of self-respect and respect for others. You can communicate your boundaries verbally by being direct yet polite. For instance, if a friend tends to borrow your things without asking, you might say, "I value our friendship, and I also value my personal belongings. I'd appreciate it if you asked me before using them." Role-playing scenarios with a friend or family member can be a helpful way to practice these conversations. Write down what you want to say before-hand to help clarify your thoughts and ensure your message is clear.

Digital Boundaries

In today's connected world, setting digital boundaries is also essential. This includes managing your time online, which platforms you use, and what personal information you share. It's also about knowing when and how to disconnect to protect your mental health. For instance, you might not check social media after nine p.m. to ensure it doesn't inter-fere with your sleep. Alternatively, keep specific details of your personal life private, sharing them only with close friends rather than broadly on social media. Setting these boundaries can help you use digital tools in a way that supports your well-being instead of undermining it. Addi-tionally, using privacy settings effectively on social platforms can help you control who sees your information and inter-acts with you, adding an extra layer of boundary that can protect against digital exhaustion and maintain healthy rela-tionships.

Navigating the complexities of personal and digital spaces requires a clear understanding of your boundaries and the confidence to assert them. By identifying, communicating, and enforcing these boundaries, you create a safe space for yourself offline and online, which is essential for your mental health and overall well-being. Remember, you have the right to protect your space and peace; setting boundaries is a powerful way to do so.

10.4 How to Ask for Help: Approaching Family and Friends

It's a familiar scene: You're feeling overwhelmed, but the thought of reaching out for help brings a pang of anxiety. You wonder if your friends or family will think you're overreacting, or that you're weak. These fears are not uncommon, but they stem from common misconceptions about what it means to seek help.

In reality, asking for support is a sign of strength and self-awareness. It shows a commitment to your well-being and trust in your cultivated relationships. Overcoming the barriers to asking for help starts with changing your perspective. Recognize that everyone needs help sometimes, and those who care about you would likely prefer you turn to them rather than struggle alone. Addressing these fears directly can diminish their power over you, freeing you to seek the support you need.

Communicating Effectively

When you decide to reach out, effective communication is critical. It's about expressing your needs clearly and confidently. Start by choosing the right time and setting. This might mean waiting for a quiet moment when the person you're approaching isn't preoccupied or stressed. Begin the conversation with an appreciation for their time or past support, which sets a positive tone. Use specific, direct phrases like, "I've been feeling overwhelmed with school lately and could use someone to talk to. Do you have time to chat?" This straightforward approach lets the other person know exactly how they can help. Avoid vague statements like "I'm just so stressed," which might not convey the seriousness of your feelings, or how they might assist you. Preparing what you want to say beforehand can help you communicate more effectively, ensuring your message is clear and your needs are understood.

Show Vulnerability

Embracing vulnerability plays a crucial role in these interactions. Opening up about your struggles can seem daunting because it exposes you to potential judgment or rejection. However, showing your vulnerable side can strengthen your relationships. It invites others to understand your experiences and emotions deeper, fostering empathy and connection. When you share your challenges, you might find that others open up about their struggles, which can deepen the bonds you share and expand your support network. Remember, being vulnerable doesn't mean sharing everything with everyone. It's about being selective and intentional with whom you choose to open up, ensuring it's someone you trust, and who has your best interests at heart.

Create a Support Plan

Creating a support plan involves a bit of strategy. This plan outlines whom to approach for help, what you'll say, and how you'll handle potential responses. Here's how to get started:

- **List Supportive People**: Write down the names of people in your life who have been supportive in the past or those you feel comfortable with.
- **Plan Your Conversation**: Script out what you want to discuss. You don't have to follow it word-for-word, but having a clear idea can ease anxiety and make the interaction smoother.
- **Consider Possible Reactions**: Think about how you'll respond to different reactions. If someone is less receptive than you hoped, plan to thank them for their time and consider who else you might approach.
- **Have a Backup Plan**: Ensure you have options if your first attempt doesn't go as expected. Having a backup plan can give you confidence and make you feel more prepared.

By creating a support plan, you can approach conversations with a clear strategy, making it easier to get the help and support you need.

In essence, asking for help is a skill that takes practice, courage, and some preparation. By addressing your fears, communicating clearly, embracing vulnerability, and having a thoughtful support plan, you empower yourself to handle life's challenges more effectively. This not only lightens your load but also strengthens your relationships, making them richer and more supportive. As you navigate the ups and downs of adolescence and beyond, remember that reaching out for help isn't just about tackling immediate problems—it's about building a support network that will be there for you throughout your life.

10.5 Healthy Romantic Relationships: A Teen's Guide

Navigating romantic relationships can sometimes feel like trying to solve a complex puzzle, where the pieces are your emotions, expectations, and experiences. Knowing which pieces fit together can create a picture of a healthy, fulfilling relationship. In contrast, forcing the wrong pieces together might lead to frustration and emotional distress. Understanding the characteristics of healthy versus unhealthy relationships is crucial in determining whether a romantic bond helps you grow or holds you back.

Characteristics of Healthy vs. Unhealthy Relationships

A healthy romantic relationship is built on mutual respect, trust, and honesty. Respect in a relationship means valuing each other's feelings, wishes, and rights. It involves appreciating each other not just for what you do but for who you are, and it manifests in actions like listening attentively, speaking kindly, and enjoying each other's differences. Trust, the cornerstone of any significant relationship, involves believing your partner will act in the relationship's best interest and not just their own. It makes you feel secure and comfortable, fostering an environment where both partners can thrive. Honesty, which ties closely with trust, involves being truthful and transparent with each other, even when the truth is complicated to say.

In stark contrast, unhealthy relationships often involve control, manipulation, and disrespect. Control can appear in various forms, such as dictating who you can spend time with, how you spend your money, or even how you dress. Manipulation, another red flag, involves using emotions or information to influence your decisions, often making you do things that are not in your best interest, or that you wouldn't do otherwise. Disrespect in relationships can be overt, like verbal abuse, or subtle, like constant criticism or chronic unreliability. Recognizing these signs can alert you to the need for change, whether addressing the issues or stepping away from the relationship.

Communicating Needs and Boundaries

Effective communication is the lifeblood of any healthy relationship, especially when expressing needs and setting boundaries. Clear communication about what you need and expect in a relationship is essential to avoid misunderstandings and to build a strong connection. Start by being straightforward about your feelings, desires, and concerns. Instead of expecting your partner to guess what you need or how you feel, express yourself clearly. Remember "I" statements? They can help focus on your feelings without placing blame.

Set and Maintain Boundaries

Setting boundaries is equally important. Boundaries help define what you are comfortable with and how you would like to be treated by others. They can be about anything that matters to you—your time, energy, and personal space. Communicate your boundaries clearly to your partner without apology. For instance, if you decide you need time to yourself, you might say, "I value our time together, but I also need time to pursue my interests." Having boundaries is not a sign of a lack of trust or love. Instead, it signifies a deep understanding of your self-worth and needs.

Dealing with Breakups

At the end of a relationship, especially your first serious one, you can feel like the floor has dropped from under you. Breakups can trigger intense emotions like sadness, anger, confusion, and relief, all mixed into a jumbled mess that can be difficult to sort through, particularly in the immediate aftermath. It's essential to allow yourself to feel these emotions without judgment. Process your feelings through healthy outlets like talking to trusted friends, writing in a journal, or engaging in physical activities. This emotional processing is crucial for healing.

Regaining self-esteem after a breakup involves reconnecting with your intrinsic worth independent of your relationship status. Engage in activities that reinforce your strengths and passions. Whether art, music, sports, or volunteering, focus on what makes you feel competent and valued. This focus can help rebuild your sense of self-worth and confidence.

Balancing Romance and Personal Growth

While romantic relationships can be essential to life, they should not be your whole life. Maintaining your individuality and pursuing your goals and interests while in a relationship is vital. Encourage each other to grow and pursue independent interests. Support each other's goals and celebrate each other's accomplishments. This mutual support strengthens the relationship and ensures that you both can grow as individuals.

Healthy romantic relationships are partnerships in which people feel valued, respected, and supported. Understanding and practicing these principles can help you build relationships that are not only joyful and loving but also empowering and enriching. As you continue to explore the world of romantic relationships, keep these guidelines in mind to help steer your interactions toward healthy dynamics that promote mutual growth and respect.

10.6 Finding Mentorship and Guidance

When you think about your path to personal and emotional growth, imagine having a guide—someone who knows the ropes, has navigated similar challenges, and can offer wisdom and support as you forge your way. This is the role of a mentor. In the vast landscape of adolescence, where every turn and dip can seem daunting, having a mentor is like having a trusted guide, who can help you navigate through. Mentors extend beyond teachers and parents.

They are coaches, family friends, or professionals, who take a genuine interest in your personal and emotional development. Their guidance can be a transformative force, providing knowledge, emotional support, and encouragement.

The Role of Mentors in Personal Development

Mentors play a crucial role in shaping your journey. They're the sounding boards for your ideas and the supportive push you need when challenges seem overwhelming. A mentor's job is to guide, inspire, and challenge you, helping you grow beyond what you think are your limits. They provide a safe space to explore your thoughts and fears without judgment, offering advice based on their experiences. This relationship can significantly boost your personal development by giving you insights into your potential and capabilities, often revealing paths and possibilities you might not have considered.

Finding the Right Mentor

Finding a mentor might seem like looking for a needle in a haystack, but it starts with knowing where to look and what criteria to consider. Start within your existing network— teachers, coaches, or leaders in your community, who have already shown interest in your development, could be potential mentors. Look for empathy, a genuine interest in helping others grow, and a career or life path that aligns with your interests. Professionals in fields you're passionate about can also be invaluable, offering guidance and a real-world connection to the careers or goals to which you aspire. When choosing a mentor, consider their availability and willingness to invest time in helping you, as a genuine mentoring relationship requires ongoing interaction and commitment.

Fostering a Mentor-Mentee Relationship

A healthy mentor-mentee relationship is built on mutual respect and a shared commitment to your growth. Establishing this relationship involves clear communication from the start. Discuss your goals, what you hope to gain from the mentoring, and what you expect from each other. Setting these expectations early helps ensure both parties are aligned and committed.

Frequent communication is critical—regular meetings, whether virtual or in-person, help maintain the connection and provide consistent support. As a mentee, be open to feedback, even when it challenges you, and be proactive in seeking advice or discussing challenges you face. A mentor is there to guide, not to handhold, so taking initiative in your growth is crucial.

Learning from Mentors

Learning with a mentor should be dynamic. Be open to their feedback and guidance, but also actively engage by asking questions, seeking clarification, and discussing how to apply their advice to real-life situations. Use what you learn to tackle personal and academic challenges and share your experiences with your mentor. This helps deepen your understanding and shows your mentor the impact of their guidance, building a mutually rewarding relationship.

Mentors are more than just advisors—they're catalysts for change. They bring a wealth of knowledge, life experiences, and insights that can greatly enrich your journey. By choosing the right mentor, building a respectful relationship, and actively participating in the process, you gain a powerful tool for personal and emotional growth. As you go through adolescence, you don't have to do it alone. A mentor can guide you, making the journey not just easier, but also more enlightening.

10.7 Effective Communication with Teachers and Peers

Navigating school life involves much more than acing tests and completing homework. It's about interacting effectively with teachers and peers—a skill that can significantly enhance your educational experience and personal relationships. Effective communication is the cornerstone of these interactions, involving more than just talking. It's about clearly exchanging ideas and actively listening. When you communicate effectively, you can clearly express your thoughts and concerns and understand others' perspectives, creating a foundation for mutual respect and understanding.

Basics of Effective Communication

At its core, effective communication involves several vital components:

- **Active Listening**: This means genuinely paying attention to what the other person is saying without planning your response while they're talking. It helps you understand their perspective and respond more thoughtfully.
- **Non-Verbal Cues**: Your body language, eye contact, and tone of voice convey a lot about your attitude and emotions. Being aware of these can help ensure that your non-verbal signals match your words, avoiding misunderstandings.
- **Clarity and Conciseness**: Being clear and concise in your verbal exchanges can prevent confusion. It's about making your point directly yet respectfully, which is especially important in a school environment where clarity and respect are essential.

Advocating for Oneself

You'll often need to advocate for yourself in school, whether asking for help with a tricky subject, negotiating a deadline extension, or discussing accommodations for learning difficulties. Start by clearly identifying your needs—what exactly do you need help with, and why? Once clear, approach the teacher at a suitable time, perhaps after class or during office hours, when you can have their full attention. Express your needs clearly and respectfully, using "I" statements to make it personal and direct, such as, "I need some guidance with this topic because I want to understand it fully." Remember, teachers are there to help you succeed, and expressing your needs clearly helps them do their job better.

Conflict Resolution Techniques

Conflicts with peers are almost inevitable, but they don't have to escalate into lasting issues. Effective conflict resolution involves negotiation and empathy. Start by expressing your perspective clearly and listening to the other person's point of view. Look for common ground or mutual interests that can serve as a basis for agreement. Then, try to negotiate a solution that benefits both sides. This might mean compromising on some points, but the goal is to resolve the conflict in a way that respects both parties' needs. Empathy is crucial here. It involves trying to understand the other person's feelings and viewpoint, which can defuse tension and lead to more constructive interactions.

Building Positive Relationships

Building and maintaining positive relationships with peers and teachers benefits your emotional and academic growth. Regular, honest communication is vital. This means talking about schoolwork or surface-level topics and sharing your thoughts and feelings when appropriate. Show genuine interest in others' lives and ideas, which can foster mutual respect and understanding. Active participation in class and school activities can also strengthen your relationships. It shows your commitment and can lead to more interactions, which help deepen connections. Always approach interactions with respect and kindness, as these values are reciprocated and form the basis of solid and positive relationships.

In this chapter, we've explored the vital role relationships play in our emotional well-being and personal growth. We've learned how to cultivate supportive friendships, set healthy boundaries, and navigate the challenges of peer pressure and bullying. We've discovered the importance of effective communication in all our relationships, from family and friends to romantic partners and mentors. We've also explored how to ask for help when needed and build positive relationships with teachers and peers. Remember, healthy relationships are built on mutual respect, trust, and clear communication.

By applying these principles and techniques, you can create a strong support network that enhances your resilience, boosts your confidence, and contributes to your overall emotional well-being. As you continue to grow and develop, these relationship skills will serve you well in all aspects of your life.

Chapter 11
Advanced Coping Strategies

I
magine playing a complex video game, where each level tests your reflexes and ability to strategize and adapt. Now, imagine if you had a unique tool that could help you understand the patterns of the game, enabling you to predict challenges and recalibrate your strategies on the fly. Cognitive Behavioral Therapy (CBT) offers a similar toolkit for navigating the complexities of your emotional and psychological world. It doesn't just help you manage your reactions but empowers you to understand and reshape them. This chapter delves into the basics of CBT, tailored specifically for you, to tackle common adolescent challenges like school stress, self-esteem issues, and social anxiety.

11.1 Introduction to Cognitive Behavioral Therapy (CBT) for Teens

Cognitive Behavioral Therapy (CBT) is a form of psychological treatment that has been extensively researched and validated by mental health professionals. It is based on the concept that your thoughts, feelings, and behaviors are interconnected, and that altering one can significantly influence others. The core principle of CBT is identifying negative or false beliefs and systematically challenging them to change unwanted behavior patterns or treat mood disorders like depression and anxiety, which are particularly prevalent during teenage years.

CBT is structured, goal-oriented, and focuses on immediate problems. It empowers you to become your own therapist with practical techniques that help you tackle your issues. Learning CBT techniques gives you an arsenal of tools to deconstruct and rebuild your thought patterns. You learn to recognize the triggers that make you feel stressed or down, dissect the validity of these triggers, and reshape your perspective to respond more positively and productively.

CBT Techniques for Teens

One of the central techniques in CBT is cognitive restructuring, which involves identifying and disputing irrational or maladaptive thoughts known as cognitive distortions. These distortions could include 'black-and-white thinking' (seeing everything at extremes without middle ground), 'overgeneralizing' (viewing a single adverse event as a never-ending pattern of defeat), or 'catastrophizing' (exaggerating the implications of an unpleasant event). By challenging these distortions, you can reduce their impact on your emotions and behaviors.

11.2 Behavioral Activation

Behavioral activation is a therapeutic technique designed to help individuals combat depression and anxiety by encouraging them to engage more fully with their environment and activities. This approach is based on the idea that our actions can significantly influence our emotions. When you're feeling depressed, you might withdraw from activities that usually bring you joy or satisfaction, creating a cycle of inactivity that deepens feelings of depression and isolation. Behavioral activation aims to break this cycle by encouraging you to participate in enjoyable or meaningful activities, which can help boost your mood and foster a sense of accomplishment.

What Is Behavioral Activation?

Behavioral activation involves identifying activities that align with your values and interests, then gradually incorporating them into your daily routine. These activities can range from simple, everyday tasks to more complex and rewarding pursuits. The key is to choose activities that you find enjoyable or meaningful, as these are more likely to have a positive impact on your mood.

How Is Behavioral Activation Done?

1. Identify Activities:

Start by making a list of activities you enjoy or used to enjoy before feeling depressed. These can include hobbies, social interactions, physical activities, or even simple tasks like taking a walk or reading a book.

Think about activities that align with your values and long-term goals. For example, if you value creativity, consider activities like drawing or writing. If social connections are important, think about reaching out to friends or joining a club.

2. Set Realistic Goals:

Begin with small, achievable goals. If you're feeling particularly low, even the smallest tasks can seem daunting. Break activities down into manageable steps. For instance, if you enjoy reading but can't focus, start with reading just a page or two.

Gradually increase the complexity and duration of these activities as you start to feel more comfortable and capable.

3. Create a Schedule:

Plan your activities ahead of time and incorporate them into your daily routine. Having a structured schedule can help you stay committed and provide a sense of purpose and direction.

Use a planner or a digital calendar to set reminders for these activities, ensuring you allocate time for them each day

4. Track Your Progress:

Keep a journal to record your activities, your level of engagement, and how you feel before and after completing them. This can help you see patterns and recognize which activities have the most positive impact on your mood.

Tracking progress also provides a sense of accomplishment, reinforcing the benefits of staying active and engaged.

5. Overcome Barriers:

Identify potential obstacles that might prevent you from engaging in activities and develop strategies to overcome them. This could include dealing with negative thoughts, finding ways to motivate yourself, or seeking support from friends or family.

Be kind to yourself if you encounter setbacks. It's normal to have days when you don't feel up to doing much. The important thing is to keep trying and gradually build up your activity level.

6. Seek Support:

Behavioral activation can be more effective with the support of a therapist or counselor who can help you identify suitable activities, set realistic goals, and provide encouragement and guidance throughout the process.

Involve friends or family members in your activities when possible. Social support can enhance the positive effects of behavioral activation and provide additional motivation.

Benefits of Behavioral Activation

- **Improved Mood:** Engaging in enjoyable activities can directly boost your mood and reduce feelings of depression.
- **Increased Motivation:** As you start to feel better, you'll likely find it easier to engage in other activities, creating a positive feedback loop.
- **Sense of Accomplishment:** Completing tasks and achieving goals, no matter how small, can provide a sense of accomplishment and improve your self-esteem.
- **Enhanced Social Connections:** Participating in social activities can help reduce feelings of isolation and build supportive relationships.
- **Breaks the Cycle of Inactivity:** By encouraging active engagement with your environment, behavioral activation helps break the cycle of inactivity and withdrawal that often accompanies depression.

In essence, behavioral activation is about taking small, manageable steps to re-engage with life. By actively participating in activities that bring joy and satisfaction, you can disrupt the negative patterns of depression and build a more positive, fulfilling routine.

11.3 Applying CBT to Common Teen Issues

Let's apply these CBT principles to scenarios in which you might find yourself. Consider school stress a common source of anxiety for many teens. Using CBT, you first identify the thoughts contributing to your stress, such as "I must always get perfect grades." You challenge this thought by evaluating its realism and helpfulness and then reframe it to something more balanced, like, "It's great to aim high, but everyone has off days, and one grade won't define my future." This cognitive restructuring helps reduce the emotional burden you might feel around schoolwork.

Self-Esteem

For issues like low self-esteem, CBT works by helping you identify negative self-talk and replace it with affirmations that promote a positive and realistic view of your capabilities. If you often think, "I'm not good at anything," CBT techniques would encourage you to list your past successes, however small, and use these to counteract the negative thoughts.

Social Anxiety

Social anxiety is another area where CBT can be incredibly effective. It teaches you to experiment with social interactions in a gradual, structured way, helping you build confidence in your social skills. You learn to manage the fear of judgment by slowly exposing yourself to social situations, assessing the reality of adverse outcomes, and practicing new ways of thinking about and engaging in social interactions.

Integration

By integrating these CBT techniques into your daily life, you learn to manage difficult emotions and situations more effectively and build a robust framework for understanding and improving your mental health. This proactive approach equips you to handle current challenges and prepares you to face future hurdles with resilience and confidence.

In this chapter, we've explored advanced coping strategies like Cognitive Behavioral Therapy (CBT) and behavioral activation, which provide practical tools for navigating the emotional and psychological challenges of adolescence. By understanding and reshaping your thoughts, engaging in activities that bring joy, and applying these techniques to real-life scenarios such as school stress, low self-esteem, and social anxiety, you can build a resilient mindset and improve your overall well-being. These strategies empower you to manage current challenges and equip you with the skills to face future hurdles confidently, fostering a healthier, more balanced approach to life.

Chapter 12
Cognitive Behavioral Techniques

Imagine you're navigating a maze, and each turn is shaped by your thoughts, leading you either to a dead end or the exit. Some of these thoughts are like funhouse mirrors, distorting your perception of reality. Cognitive Behavioral Therapy (CBT) gives you a map and compass to spot these distortions and find your way through the mental maze more effectively. This chapter dives into one key aspect of CBT: understanding cognitive distortions —those misleading thoughts that can deeply impact your emotions and behaviors.' 12.1 Understanding Cognitive Distortions

Cognitive distortions are like optical illusions for the mind, convincing us of things that aren't true. These irrational thought patterns can warp our perception of reality, leading to negative emotions and unhelpful behaviors. For example, 'all-or-nothing thinking' might make you feel like a complete failure if you're not perfect in school. 'Overgeneralization' might lead you to believe that if something goes wrong once, it will always go wrong. Another common distortion is 'catastrophizing,' where you expect disaster no matter the situation, like assuming one bad grade will ruin your entire academic career.

Impact

These distortions can profoundly impact your behavior and emotions. For example, if you constantly engage in 'all-or-nothing thinking,' you might avoid trying new activities where you expect you can't excel, leading to missed opportunities and feelings of sadness or inadequacy. Overgeneralizing from a single negative experience can result in broader anxiety and avoidance behaviors, limiting your experiences and personal growth. Catastrophizing can keep you in a perpetual state of stress and panic, affecting your physical health and overall well-being.

Pattern Recognition

Recognizing these patterns is the first step toward change. To spot these distortions in your everyday life, closely observe your reactions to various situations. When you feel upset or behave in a way that seems out of proportion, pause and reflect. What was going through my mind just now? Write down these thoughts and look for patterns. See if you can categorize these thoughts under the common cognitive distortions. This exercise can be eye-opening, revealing how often distorted thinking influences your mood and actions.

Build Awareness

Building awareness of cognitive distortions is crucial. It's mapping out the maze—understanding the walls and barriers in your thinking. Awareness alone can sometimes reduce the power of these distortions. By continually monitoring your thoughts and identifying distortions, you gradually train your brain to recognize and rectify these patterns automatically. This self-monitoring is a powerful tool in your mental toolkit that empowers you to navigate your thoughts more effectively, enhancing your ability to manage stress, build relationships, and face life's challenges with a clearer, more balanced perspective.

Integration

Incorporating these techniques into your daily routine might seem challenging at first, but like any new skill, it becomes easier with practice. Start small with a daily journaling habit. Spend a few minutes each evening reflecting on your thoughts and emotions and identify any cognitive distortions you encountered. This simple practice can reveal how your thoughts affect your feelings and behaviors, leading to deeper insights and changes in your thought patterns. As you get better at recognizing and adjusting these distortions, you'll find it easier to navigate your mind and achieve a healthier mental state.' 12.2 Developing Counterstatements for Negative Thoughts

Imagine you're in a debate, and every time you make a point, there's an opposing view trying to overshadow your argument. Now, think of your mind as where negative thoughts often take the microphone, spreading doubt and pessimism. Developing counterstatements is like preparing yourself with solid and evidence-based rebuttals that neutralize these pervasive negative thoughts. This technique is a cornerstone of Cognitive Behavioral Therapy (CBT) and involves examining the evidence for and against distorted thoughts, replacing them with more balanced, rational alternatives.

Technique of Counterstatements

Let's break down the process: Say you're faced with the thought, "I'll never be good at math." This is a typical example of 'all-or-nothing' thinking. To develop a counterstatement, you must first challenge this thought by looking for evidence that contradicts it. Have there been times when you've done well in math? Can you think of occasions when you've solved a complex problem, or scored higher than expected? List these instances as evidence against the negative thought. Next, craft a balanced counterstatement like, "While math is challenging for me, I have succeeded in several assignments and can improve with practice and help." This response is not overly optimistic but is realistic and supportive, reducing the emotional weight of the original negative thought. Practice Through Scenarios

Consider a scenario where you feel overwhelmed by a big project. You might think, "This is impossible. I can't manage this." To flip this thought, you could break down the project into smaller, manageable tasks and remind yourself of past projects you've successfully completed. A counterstatement could be, "I've handled challenging projects before by organizing them into smaller tasks, and I can do the same this time." Using structured templates or worksheets, jot down these scenarios and practice writing counterstatements for each. Regular practice can turn this into a quick, almost automatic response in real-life situations.

Long-Term Benefits

Engaging regularly in this practice can dramatically shift your mental landscape. One of the most significant benefits is increased self-esteem. Each time you counter a negative thought, you affirm your abilities and reduce self-doubt, gradually building a more positive self-image. Moreover, better decision-making comes from seeing situations more clearly and realistically, without the distortion of negative biases. Improved emotional regulation is another crucial benefit, as you're less likely to be swayed by extreme emotions tied to inaccurate thoughts. This skill helps maintain emotional balance, especially in challenging situations.

Encouragement for Regular Practice

Integrate this technique into your daily routine:

- Integrate your thinking patterns.
- Set aside a few minutes each day for reflection—perhaps in the evening—to review moments when negative thoughts arose.
- Write these down and develop counterstatements for each.

This practice builds strength against negative thinking and enhances your ability to approach life's challenges with a more balanced and proactive mindset. Like any skill, the more you practice, the more proficient you become. So, keep at it, and watch as your mind learns to support rather than sabotage your efforts, opening up a world where challenges are just undiscovered opportunities.

12.3 The ABC Model: Breaking Down Emotional Reactions

Imagine you're walking through your school hallway, and a classmate bumps into you out of nowhere, spilling your books everywhere. Your immediate thought might be, "They did that on purpose." This thought sparks anger, leading you to react, perhaps by shouting or storming off in frustration. This scenario is a textbook example of the ABC model in Cognitive Behavioral Therapy (CBT), where A stands for Antecedent (the event), B for Belief (your thought about the event), and C for Consequence (your emotional and behavioral reaction). The ABC model helps you dissect these moments to understand better how your interpretations of events influence your feelings and actions.

Explanation of the ABC Model

The ABC model is a framework used in CBT to illustrate how your beliefs about a situation affect how you react emotionally and behaviorally. 'A' is the Antecedent, the actual event and the immediate trigger for your response; 'B' is your Belief about the event, which involves your interpretation or perception of what happened; and 'C' is the Consequence, which includes your emotional, psychological, and physical response to the event. This model teaches that while you might not always have control over the Antecedent, you can learn to identify and adjust your beliefs, which can significantly change the consequences.

Application in Everyday Situations

To apply the ABC model in daily life, identify a recent event that triggered a strong emotional reaction. For instance, consider a time when you received a lower grade than expected on a test. That's your Antecedent. Your Belief might be, "I'm terrible at this subject," leading to feelings of discouragement or failure (the Consequence). By dissecting this event through the ABC model, you can begin to see how changing your Belief—for example, to "I didn't do well this time, but I can learn from my mistakes and improve"—could alter your emotional response helping you feel more motivated rather than defeated.

Interactive Examples

Let's try mapping out the ABCs for a typical teenage stressor: peer conflict. Imagine you text a friend to hang out, and they reply only for a few hours. The Antecedent is the friend not replying. If your Belief is "They're ignoring me because they don't like me," the Consequence might be feeling rejected and sad, leading you to avoid your friend. However, if you adjust your Belief to "They might be busy or haven't seen my message," your emotional response might be more understanding and patient, leading to a more positive interaction once you connect.

Strategies to Alter Beliefs

Altering your beliefs takes practice and involves challenging the accuracy of your automatic thoughts. By questioning and adjusting your beliefs, you can start to influence the emotional and behavioral consequences in a way that's more in line with how you want to feel and react. Here's how to do it.

Identify a negative belief and ask yourself:

- "Is this thought based on facts or assumptions?"
- "Are there alternative explanations?"

Example: Worrying about participating in class:

- Negative Belief: "Everyone will think I'm stupid if I get this wrong."
- Questions to Challenge It:
- "Could it be that others are too focused on their own participation to judge mine?"
- Alternative Belief: "Everyone makes mistakes, and that's okay."

By changing your belief, you can reduce anxiety and feel more encouraged to participate in class.

By consistently applying the ABC model, you equip your-self with a powerful tool to understand and manage how you interpret and react to the world around you. This skill enhances your ability to handle challenging situations and empowers you to create a more positive and fulfilling emotional life. It's not the events themselves but your beliefs about them that often shape your emotions.

12.4 Dialectical Behavior Therapy (DBT) Skills You Can Use

Dialectical Behavior Therapy, commonly known as DBT, is designed to help people manage overwhelming emotions and improve their interpersonal relationships. Originally developed to treat borderline personality disorder, DBT has proven effective for a wide range of emotional and psycho-logical issues. At its core, DBT focuses on providing you with skills to cope with stress, control your emotions, and improve your relationships with others. Unlike other thera-pies that focus solely on analysis, DBT is skill-based, putting a strong emphasis on practical strategies to manage emotional distress and enhance communication.

Core DBT Skills

DBT is built around four primary skills, each designed to address specific emotional and interpersonal challenges:

- **Mindfulness**: The foundation of all DBT skills. It involves learning to live in the moment and accept things as they are without judgment. This skill helps you become more aware of your thoughts and feelings, reducing reactions driven by emotional ups and downs.

- **Distress Tolerance**: Essential for managing overwhelming emotions. It teaches you to tolerate and survive crises without resorting to self-destructive behaviors.
- **Emotional Regulation**: Provides strategies to manage and change intense emotions that cause problems in your life.
- **Interpersonal Effectiveness**: Equips you with techniques to assert your needs and wants while maintaining positive relationships and self-respect.

DBT Exercises for Daily Life

To integrate DBT skills into your daily routine:

- **Start with simple mindfulness exercises**: Try "Wise Mind" practices. A Wise Mind is the balanced part of you that combines your emotional and reasonable sides. It helps you make logically sound decisions while tuning into your emotions. An exercise to access your Wise Mind could involve focusing on your breath and asking yourself, "What is wise for me now?" Regular practice can help you develop a centered mind, especially in stressful situations.

- **Reality acceptance skills**: Use these for moments when you can't change a distressing situation. Techniques like "turning the mind" involve consciously accepting reality as it is. This can reduce the pain of resistance and open a pathway to emotional healing.
- **Coping cards**: These are handy tools for dealing with difficult emotions on the go. These small cards list coping statements or reminders to help you manage emotions or resist impulsive behaviors.

Integrating DBT into Social Interactions

DBT can dramatically improve how you interact with people. The skills you learn can help you communicate more clearly, assert your needs, manage conflicts without damaging your relationships, and even strengthen your relationships. For instance, learning to express your feelings and needs directly using clear statements can help reduce misunderstandings and conflicts with friends and family.

Role-playing different scenarios with a friend or therapist can be a great way to practice these skills. For example, you could practice asking a friend to return a borrowed item using precise, respectful communication techniques. DBT also emphasizes the importance of negotiation and compromise, which are vital in maintaining relationships even when conflicts arise. By practicing these skills, you can enhance your ability to maintain healthier, more satisfying relationships and lead a happier, more balanced life.

Integrating DBT skills into your daily routines and social interactions allows you to gain greater control over your emotions and build better relationships, paving the way for a more fulfilling and balanced life. As you continue to practice these skills, you're likely able to handle emotional challenges more effectively, improve your communication, and deepen your connections with others. Remember, like any set of skills, proficiency comes with practice and persistence. Keep at it. Over time, you'll see significant changes in how you manage your emotions and interact with the world around you.

12.5 Mastering Emotional Regulation with DBT

Emotional regulation might sound like a heavy term. Still, in the context of DBT (Dialectical Behavior Therapy), it's about managing those intense emotions that can suddenly overwhelm you, making it hard to think clearly or react reasonably. It's like being in the driver's seat of your emotional car—without regulation, it's as though your car is speeding down a steep hill without brakes. DBT provides the techniques to install these brakes and use them effectively, ensuring you maintain control even when emotions try to take the wheel.

Emotions Are Not Your Enemy

Understanding emotional regulation within DBT involves recognizing that emotions are not your enemies. They are messengers that alert you to what's happening internally and externally. However, when these emotions become too intense, they can lead to distress, impulsive actions, and even long-term problems like anxiety or depression. DBT teaches you to reduce the frequency and intensity of these overwhelming emotions by increasing your awareness of them, understanding their triggers, and learning to manage them through specific skills and exercises.

Identify Triggers

Explicitly identifying what triggers your intense emotions is a crucial step. This might be stress from upcoming exams, conflicts with friends, or internal pressures like self-criticism. Using DBT worksheets or diaries to track these triggers can be incredibly insightful. You would note down situations where intense emotions arise and describe what was happening, what thoughts went through your mind, and how you reacted. Over time, patterns will emerge, showing you the most common triggers, and your typical responses to them. This awareness is your first tool in emotional regulation, as it allows you to anticipate and prepare for challenging situations.

Practical Skills

DBT offers several practical skills for emotional regulation, one of which is the 'opposite action' technique. This skill is about doing the exact opposite of what your emotional urges tell you to do, provided these urges aren't aligned with your rational goals or values. For example, if you feel the urge to isolate yourself when sad, the opposite action would be to reach out to a friend or join a family activity. This technique is based on the idea that changing your actions can change your emotions, breaking the cycle of negative feelings and leading to negative behaviors, reinforcing negative feelings.

Real-Life Scenarios

Let's explore how you apply DBT skills in real-life scenarios to enhance your ability to regulate emotions. Imagine facing a common teenage scenario of receiving criticism from a teacher in front of your classmates. Your immediate reaction might be embarrassment or anger, and your urge might be to retort sharply or completely disengage. However, by applying the 'opposite action' technique, you would instead choose to respond calmly by asking constructive questions about how you can improve, or simply thanking the teacher for the feedback. This response helps manage your emotions at the moment and builds your resilience and ability to handle criticism constructively in the future.

Regular practice of these skills is critical to mastering emotional regulation. Understanding them theoretically is one thing, but the real benefits come through consistent application in everyday situations. Start using a DBT diary to track your emotions and triggers daily. As you become more comfortable with the techniques, you'll react more effectively at the moment and begin to experience less intense negative feelings over time. This process enhances your overall emotional stability and well-being, empowering you to navigate the complexities of teenage life with confidence and calm.

12.6 Distress Tolerance: Techniques for Tough Times

Imagine you're in a situation that feels like the emotional equivalent of being stuck in a traffic jam on a hot day with no air conditioning. The frustration builds, the heat rises, and everything feels ten times more intense. Distress tolerance is about finding ways to roll down the windows, turn on some music, and make the situation more bearable until you can move again. In the realm of Dialectical Behavior Therapy (DBT), developing distress tolerance is crucial for those moments when emotions run high and the usual coping mechanisms just don't cut it.

Distress tolerance involves skills to help you withstand and manage acute emotional distress without resorting to harmful behaviors. These skills are precious when you are in situations you cannot change immediately or when your emotions become overwhelming. The goal isn't to eliminate distress—that's not always possible—but to endure it without escalating the situation or hurting yourself or others.

Crisis Survival Strategies

One of the most practical aspects of distress tolerance is learning crisis survival strategies. You can use immediate tools and techniques to help you through challenging moments without worsening things.

Distraction

Distraction is one such strategy. It's about intentionally diverting your attention from distressing emotions and focusing on something more neutral or positive. This could be anything from watching a favorite comedy show to diving into a graphic novel or playing a video game. The key is to choose activities that are absorbing enough to provide a temporary break from distress.

Self-Soothing

Self-soothing is another powerful strategy. It's all about comforting yourself through your senses. Creating a playlist of songs that lift your mood, lighting a calming candle, or wrapping up in a soft blanket are all examples of self-soothing. It's about doing minor, nurturing things that help calm and comfort your nervous system.

Visualization

Improving the moment involves techniques to make your current situation more bearable. Visualization can be particularly effective here. For instance, when stressed, you might close your eyes and imagine yourself in a peaceful place, like a quiet beach or a cool forest. This mental escape can provide a brief respite from reality, lowering stress levels. Another technique is relaxation breathing, where you focus on taking slow, deep breaths to help reduce tension and anxiety.

Acceptance Skills

Radical acceptance is a cornerstone of distress tolerance and involves fully accepting reality at the moment without judgment. This doesn't mean you approve of the situation, or that it isn't painful, but rather, you acknowledge it for what it is. Radical acceptance is powerful because struggling against reality often intensifies emotional turmoil. It's like being caught in quicksand—the more you struggle, the deeper you sink. By accepting the situation, you stop the struggle and find ways to cope with the pain.

Exercises for Building Distress Tolerance

Building your distress tolerance muscle is like any other form of training—it requires practice and consistency.

Diary

One helpful exercise is the distress tolerance diary, where you document episodes of distress and note which strategies you used and how effective they were. This helps you track your progress and identify which techniques work best for you in different situations.

Scenario Planning

Another exercise involves scenario planning. Here, you imagine potentially distressing situations and plan how to apply distress tolerance skills. For example, suppose you're anxious about an upcoming public speaking event. In that case, you should use self-soothing techniques beforehand, such as listening to calming music or practicing deep breathing exercises. During the event, you might use distraction by focusing on friendly faces in the audience or the content of your speech rather than your anxiety.

Practicing these distress tolerance techniques regularly can significantly improve your handling of emotional crises. They equip you with tools to manage intense feelings effectively, reducing the likelihood of engaging in self-destructive behaviors. Over time, as you become more adept at these skills, you'll find that you can navigate life's challenges with more composure, transforming what once felt like overwhelming roadblocks into manageable detours.

12.7 Interpersonal Effectiveness: Communicating Your Needs

Navigating the intricate dance of interpersonal relationships can sometimes feel like speaking a foreign language. Each interaction can have complexities, whether with friends, family, or teachers. Interpersonal effectiveness is your skill set for this dance—it involves communicating your needs and boundaries clearly and assertively, managing conflicts gracefully, and maintaining healthy relationships. It's about ensuring that your relationships are not just about getting along but also about getting what you need and want in a way that respects you and others.

DEAR MAN Strategy

Understanding interpersonal effectiveness starts with recognizing that every interaction is an opportunity to meet your objectives, including your wants, needs, or how you wish to be treated. However, effectiveness isn't just about being assertive—it's equally about maintaining relationships and self-respect. It's a balancing act. Pushing too hard can damage relationships, while not making enough can lead to resentment and unmet needs. Here, specific communication skills, such as those encapsulated in the DEAR MAN strategy, come into play. This acronym stands for Describe, Express, Assert, Reinforce, stay Mindful, Appear confident, and Negotiate. Each component serves a particular purpose:

- **Describe**: State the facts of the situation clearly, without judgment.
- **Express**: Convey your feelings and opinions about the problem.
- **Assert**: Don't be afraid to ask for what you want or say no clearly.
- **Reinforce**: Explain the positive effects of getting what you want or need.
- **(Stay) Mindful**: Keep the focus on your goals despite distractions or opposition.
- **Appear Confident**: Support your words with your manner, maintaining eye contact and an assertive posture.
- **Negotiate**: Be willing to give to get, finding a compromise where both parties can agree.

Handling Conflicts

Handling interpersonal conflicts effectively is another crucial aspect. Conflicts are inevitable in any relationship, but the fallout doesn't have to be destructive. The key is to manage disputes in ways that address the issue while preserving the relationship. This requires empathy, patience, and often, creativity.

For example, if you and a sibling are at odds over privacy boundaries in your shared room, the conflict management strategy shouldn't just be about setting strict rules. It should also consider each person's needs, and how to meet them halfway. Techniques like active listening, where you truly hear and validate the other person's perspective, and "I-statements" that express your feelings without blaming, can de-escalate conflicts and pave the way for mutual understanding and solutions.

Role-Playing

Role-playing exercises are an excellent way to practice these skills. For instance, you could simulate a scenario where you negotiate a later curfew with your parents. Start by **describing** why you feel a later curfew is reasonable, **express** how the current curfew makes you feel left out from social gatherings, **assert** what time you think would be fair, **reinforce** how this change would make you feel more trusted and responsible, remain **mindful** to keep the conversation on track, **appear** confident to show you are serious, and be ready to **negotiate,** perhaps by agreeing to certain conditions like check-in calls. Such exercises prepare you for real-life interactions, making it easier to navigate them successfully when they occur.

By mastering interpersonal effectiveness, you enhance your ability to communicate and resolve conflicts and build stronger, healthier relationships that can withstand the challenges of misunderstandings and disagreements. By continually practicing these skills, you create a repertoire of strategies that can transform your interactions, making them functional and fulfilling. As you integrate these practices into your daily interactions, notice the shift in how you and those around you respond. It's these subtle shifts that, over time, strengthen the bonds you have and foster new ones, enriching your social and emotional life.

12.8 The Art of Mindfulness in DBT

Finding a moment of quiet reflection can seem revolutionary in the bustling hallways of life, where every corner buzzes with demands and distractions. This is where Dialectical Behavior Therapy (DBT) introduces a transformative aspect of mindfulness, tailored not just to quiet the mind but to enhance your interactions and manage your emotions to align with your goals and values. Unlike general mindfulness practices that may focus broadly on awareness and presence, mindfulness in DBT is specifically fine-tuned to help you navigate the emotional high seas, keeping your ship steady even when the waters get rough.

What and How

Mindfulness in DBT is structured around two core skill sets: "What" and "How" skills. The "What" skills include observing, describing, and participating in foundational mindfulness actions. Observing involves taking note of your environment and internal state without reacting—like watching clouds pass in the sky, you notice thoughts and feelings without attaching to them. Describing adds a layer to observing by putting words to your experiences. This might mean acknowledging, "I feel anxious," rather than simply noticing a tightness in your chest. Participating allows you to fully engage in the current activity without self-consciousness, immersing yourself fully in the task, whether it's a conversation, a classroom lecture, or even a mundane chore like washing dishes.

The "How" skills—non-judgmentally, one-mindfully, and effectively—focus on how you practice these actions. Acting non-judgmentally is crucial, as it involves accepting thoughts, feelings, and sensations without criticism and, for instance, acknowledging that you feel annoyed by a friend's comment without labeling the emotion or yourself as inadequate. One-mindfully refers to doing one thing at a time, which can be profoundly influential in an era of constant multitasking. It's about listening to a song without scrolling through your phone, thoroughly absorbing, and enjoying the experience, and being effective means focusing on doing what works rather than what is "right" according to your judgments or rules dictated by others. This might involve choosing a pragmatic approach to solving a problem in a group project, even if it's not the approach you would personally prefer.

Integration

Integrating these mindfulness practices into your daily life can transform your routine and interactions. Start by setting aside a few minutes each day to practice observing your thoughts and feelings without judgment. You can do this anytime and anywhere—whether waiting for the bus or during a quiet moment before bed. Use this time to notice what's happening within and around you, letting thoughts and sensations come and go. Gradually incorporate mindfulness into daily activities. For instance, when eating, pay attention to your food's taste, texture, and smell, fully experiencing the act of eating. When speaking with someone, focus entirely on the conversation without planning what you'll say next, or thinking about your next task.

Consider a scenario where you feel incredibly anxious about an upcoming exam to see how mindfulness can be particularly effective. The typical reaction might be to spiral into worry, imagining worst-case scenarios, or to distract yourself by binge-watching a series. Instead, try using your DBT mindfulness skills. Observe your anxiety without judgment, describe the sensations and thoughts you are having, and participate fully in a calming activity like deep breathing or listening to soothing music. By focusing one-mindfully on this activity, you effectively reduce your anxiety and are better prepared to tackle your study session.

Practicing mindfulness in this DBT-specific way offers a powerful toolkit for dealing with emotional intensity and enhancing your interactions. It's about more than just surviving your teen years. It's about thriving in them, equipped with skills to experience life more fully, manage stress more effectively, and navigate your relationships with greater ease and understanding. As you continue to practice these techniques, you'll likely find that they become a natural part of your daily routine, helping you to stay centered and poised, even in the face of life's inevitable challenges.

12.9 Problem-Solving Strategies for Everyday Challenges

In a teen's life, every day can unfold like a series of puzzles, each with its own set of challenges. Whether deciding on a college major, sorting out a disagreement with a friend, or juggling a hectic schedule, the ability to solve problems effectively is crucial. This isn't just about finding quick fixes but developing a strategy that you can apply to various situations, ensuring you make thoughtful and beneficial decisions. Let's break down the steps involved in practical problem-solving, which will help you handle real-life issues more adeptly.

Problem-Solving Steps

- **The first step in any problem-solving process is to identify the problem.** This sounds straightforward, but often, situations are viewed through a lens of emotional reactions, which can cloud judgment. Take the process of choosing a college major—a decision that might seem overwhelming due to its impact on your future career and life. Start by defining what makes this choice challenging. Is it pressure from family? Uncertainty about what you're passionate about? Or concerns about job prospects? Pinpointing the specific problem helps in addressing it directly.

- **Once the problem is identified, brainstorm possible solutions.** Here, quantity trumps quality—list all possible options, even those that seem far-fetched or unconventional. For instance, solutions range from talking to career counselors and contacting professionals in your fields of interest to taking online courses to gauge your enthusiasm for the subjects.

- **The next step is to evaluate these solutions.** Consider the pros and cons of each option, and how well they align with your values, interests, and long-term goals. This might involve research or discussion with trusted advisors to gather information and perspectives.

- **Finally, please select the most suitable solution and implement it.** This step requires commitment and, sometimes, a leap of faith. It's essential to monitor the outcomes and be ready to revisit the problem-solving process if the initial solution doesn't pan out as expected.

Applying Problem-Solving to Real-Life Issues

Consider the common scenario of resolving a conflict with a friend. Let's say your friend has shared something told in confidence. Start by identifying the problem. Is it the breach of trust, or is it more about how the incident made you feel? Next, brainstorm potential ways to address it, including having an honest conversation with your friend, setting more explicit boundaries in the future, or taking time apart to reassess the friendship.

Evaluate these based on how likely they are to mend the relationship and how comfortable you feel with each approach. Please choose the best solution, act on it, and observe how it changes the dynamics of your friendship. This systematic approach provides clarity and empowers you to handle emotional situations more rationally.

Overcoming Obstacles in Problem-Solving

Problem-solving can be a challenging process'. It's common to encounter obstacles such as emotional blocks, lack of information, or external pressures. Emotional blocks, for example, can make it hard to function logically under stress. Techniques from CBT and DBT, like mindfulness and distress tolerance, can help manage these emotions, allowing you to approach problems more calmly and effectively. Lack of information can be tackled through research, asking for advice, or consulting experts. External pressures, such as expectations from parents or peers, require you to ground yourself in your values firmly and, sometimes, to communicate your needs and decisions assertively.

By mastering these problem-solving steps and learning to navigate the associated challenges, you equip yourself with a valuable skill set that applies to nearly all areas of life. From academic and personal decisions to future career paths, becoming an adept problem-solver smooths your current journey and sets you up for long-term success. As you move forward, remember that each problem solved adds to your experience, builds your confidence, and enhances your ability to face whatever comes next with resilience and poise.

In this chapter, we've explored a variety of strategies and techniques from CBT and DBT that you can apply to manage emotions, handle stress, and improve interpersonal relationships. Each tool helps in specific situations and contributes to a broader understanding of yourself and how you interact with the world. As we transition to the next chapter, we'll delve deeper into how you can continue to apply these skills in more complex scenarios, ensuring you're prepared to meet life's challenges with confidence and clarity.

Chapter 13
Preparing for Life Transitions

Imagine standing at the edge of a giant Olympic diving board. Below you, the water is clear and inviting, but the height is dizzying. Taking that leap is a lot like transitioning from high school to college. It's exciting, a little scary, and significantly changes your life. You're moving from a familiar routine and environment to a world with new challenges and opportunities. This transition isn't just about academic changes. It involves evolving your personal and emotional landscapes.

13.1 High School to College: Emotional Prep 101

Transitioning from high school to college brings a cascade of changes. You're expected to handle increased academic demands:

- The workload is heavier.
- The material is more complex.
- You often learn in large, impersonal lecture halls rather than small, interactive classes.

Beyond academics, you're also navigating a new social environment. For many of you, this will be your first time living away from home, which means new living arrangements— dorms, roommates, and a new level of personal responsibility. You're also tasked with building a new social network from scratch, an exciting but sometimes daunting task.

This period of your life is thrilling and packed with opportunities to learn and grow. However, it also comes with challenges. Managing your own schedule is exciting but can feel overwhelming. The pressure to make new friends and fit into new social circles can be intense. It's normal to feel a mix of anticipation, anxiety, excitement, and fear. Recognizing these emotions as a natural part of the transition can help you handle them more effectively.

Developing Independence

Independence is one of the major developmental milestones you'll encounter as you move into college life. Managing finances, balancing social life with academics, and making health care decisions are all part of the college experience. Developing strong time management skills is crucial. Consider using tools like digital calendars or planners to keep track of your commitments and deadlines. Financial independence is another critical area. Start by creating a simple budget to track your expenses and savings. This not only helps in managing your money but also teaches you valuable life skills in financial planning.

Decision-making is yet another aspect of independence. In college, you'll make numerous decisions daily, from minor choices. like what to eat for lunch, to major ones like choosing your major or career path. These decisions can shape your future, so think about them carefully. Trust your instincts and seek advice from trusted mentors, counselors, or family members when needed.

Emotional Readiness

While the freedom and new experiences of college life are exciting, they can also lead to feelings of homesickness and emotional stress. It's important to recognize these feelings and address them proactively. Stay connected with family and friends from home through regular calls or messages. At the same time, immerse yourself in the new experiences college offers. Engaging in campus activities, joining clubs, or volunteering can help you feel more connected to your new environment.

Seeking support when feeling overwhelmed is crucial. Most colleges provide resources like counseling centers, academic advising, and student health services. Get to know these resources early on. They can help you manage stress, tackle academic challenges, and handle serious mental health issues.

Resource Identification

As you navigate this new chapter, knowing where to find help can make all the difference. During your first weeks on campus, take the time to locate and familiarize yourself with critical resources. The counseling center can be a sanctuary for mental health support, while the academic advising office can help you plan your course load and tackle any academic issues. Health services provide medical care when needed, ensuring you don't struggle to find a doctor or pharmacy in a pinch.

Many colleges also offer workshops on stress management and study skills. Participating in these can provide you with additional tools to handle the challenges of college life. Remember, these resources are there for your benefit, so don't hesitate to use them.

Navigating the transition from high school to college is no small feat. It's a profound journey of personal and academic growth. By anticipating the challenges, developing independence, preparing emotionally, and utilizing available resources, you set the stage for a successful and enriching college experience. Every big change begins with the decision to take a step. As you dive into college life, do so with confidence and excitement, knowing you have the tools to navigate this new journey successfully.

13.2 Managing Expectations: Yours vs. Those of Others

In the whirl of daily life, especially during transitions such as moving from high school to college, it's easy to find yourself caught between what you want for yourself and what others expect of you. The expectations of parents, teachers, and friends can sometimes overshadow your own, making it challenging to stay true to your aspirations. It's like walking a tightrope, where you balance your dreams and the hopes others have placed on you. The key to maintaining this balance isn't just about meeting these expectations but integrating them with your goals in a way that still respects your individuality and personal growth.

Clarifying Personal Goals

Understanding what you want is crucial. This clarity comes from introspection—a deep dive into your desires, motivations, and values. Start by setting aside time for yourself, away from the noise and demands of everyday life. Use this time to reflect on questions like: What am I passionate about? What goals make me excited about the future? Write these thoughts down. They don't have to be perfectly formed, but they must reflect your true interests. This exercise isn't about crafting an impeccable plan for the next ten years. It's about identifying what matters to you right now, which can guide your decisions and help you set boundaries against external pressures.

Once you have a clearer idea of your goals, align them with

actionable steps. For instance, if your goal is to become a graphic designer, your steps include taking specific courses, engaging in design contests, or seeking internships. These steps should resonate with your values and interests, not just be a path laid down by external expectations.

Balancing External Expectations

Balancing your goals with others' expectations involves open communication and negotiation. For example, your parents might value job security and encourage a stable career path. If their expectations clash with your dreams, like pursuing a career in the arts, explain your passion and why it matters to you. Provide a clear plan for how you intend to pursue your career responsibly.

Communication should be clear and confident. Articulate your plans to show you've thought things through. While this might not always lead to agreement, it can foster understanding and compromise. Remember, most external expectations, especially from loved ones, come from a place of concern and wanting you to succeed. Acknowledging this can make these conversations more constructive and less confrontational.

Dealing with Pressure

Pressure to meet external expectations can often lead to stress, especially when these expectations feel at odds with personal goals. Managing this stress effectively is crucial for your mental and emotional health. Techniques such as mindfulness meditation or regular physical activity can be powerful tools for stress relief. They help clear your mind and reduce anxiety, making focusing on what truly matters easier.

Moreover, don't hesitate to seek support. Talking to mentors or peers who have faced similar pressures can provide relief and practical strategies for managing expectations. Sometimes, knowing others have navigated similar paths and succeeded can be incredibly reassuring.

Adjusting Expectations

Finally, be prepared to adjust your expectations realistically. This adjustment is not about lowering your standards or giving up on your dreams but about adapting to realities without losing sight of your goals. It's about flexible thinking —setting high but attainable goals and being open to modifying them as you gain more experience and insight.

For instance, if you find that the academic load in college is more challenging than expected, adjusting your study habits or seeking help is a practical response. This flexibility helps prevent disappointment and fosters a resilient and adaptive mindset—a mindset that sees every challenge as a learning opportunity and every setback as a chance to grow.

Navigating the maze of personal and external expectations is no small feat, but with clear goals, open communication, effective stress management, and flexible thinking, you can successfully maintain this balance. The ultimate aim is to mold a life that feels authentic to you, enriched by your experiences, and aligned with your vision of success.

13.3 Embracing New Roles and Responsibilities

Stepping into a new role, whether as a college student, a part-time employee, or simply taking on more responsibilities at home, is like updating your app version—it's still you, but with more features and perhaps a few unexpected bugs to manage. These transitions can be exhilarating, offering new freedoms and opportunities, but they can also be daunting, requiring shifts in your self-perception and responsibilities. Emotionally, this evolution can stir both excitement and anxiety as you navigate the balance between old expectations and new realities.

Prioritizing

Transitioning into new roles often brings a significant increase in responsibility. You're not just responsible for your grades anymore; you might also be managing your finances, balancing work and study, or caring for younger siblings. This increase in responsibilities can feel overwhelming. Prioritization becomes crucial in these situations. Recognize that while all responsibilities are important, they don't all require immediate attention. Learning to prioritize effectively—identifying which tasks need immediate action and which can wait—can significantly reduce the stress of juggling multiple responsibilities.

Delegation

Delegation is another crucial strategy. It's about under-standing that just because you can do something doesn't mean you always should. For instance, resist the urge to take on all tasks if you're working on a group project. Divide the work according to each member's strengths and availability. At home, family responsibilities can also be shared. Open communication about each family member's capacity and time constraints can help distribute tasks more evenly, ensuring no one is overwhelmed.

Boundaries

Setting boundaries is equally crucial. These are not just physical or emotional limits. They're also about your time and energy. It's okay to say no or to renegotiate deadlines when necessary. This isn't about forgetting responsibility but ensuring you can handle your responsibilities without burning out. For example, explaining your situation and asking for a compromise is reasonable if you're invited to take extra shifts at work during exam week.

Conflicts

Navigating role conflicts requires a blend of good time management and effective communication. For many teens, conflicts arise when school, work, and social life demands collide. You may have a part-time job that eats into your study time, or your social commitments clash with family responsibilities. Managing these conflicts often involves tough choices and trade-offs.

A helpful approach is to communicate openly with the

people involved. If work conflicts with your studies, talk to your employer about adjusting your schedule. If social activities impact your family duties, discuss these commitments with your family to find a mutually agreeable balance. Often, people are more understanding and willing to accommodate your needs when you communicate clearly and respectfully.

Self-Reflection

Self-reflection is an invaluable tool as you navigate these new roles. It involves regularly taking a step back to assess how you manage your responsibilities and adapt to your roles. Are you feeling stretched too thin? Are there commitments that no longer serve your goals or well-being? Reflective practices like journaling can be beneficial here. By writing down your experiences and feelings, you can gain insights into what's working and what isn't. This ongoing self-assessment allows you to make necessary adjustments, ensuring your roles and responsibilities evolve to support your personal development and emotional health.

Embracing new roles and responsibilities is a dynamic process filled with learning and adjustment. It's about finding what works for you, managing increased demands, and ensuring you stay in the process. With the right strategies—prioritization, delegation, setting boundaries, managing conflicts, and regular self-reflection—you can navigate these changes effectively, making the most of the new opportunities for growth and learning that these roles inevitably bring.

13.4 Coping with Failure and Rejection

Nobody cruises through life without hitting some bumps. These setbacks can sting, whether it's a bad grade, not making the team, or facing rejection from a college or job you really wanted. However, it's crucial to understand that experiencing failure and rejection is a fundamental part of human life. More importantly, these moments are not just obstacles. They can be significant catalysts for growth and self-discovery.

Learn From It

First off, think of failure and rejection as not just inevitable but as vital teachers. They are universal experiences that provide invaluable lessons about inner strength and adaptability. The key is to shift your perspective to view each setback as an opportunity to learn and evolve. For instance, a failed exam can reveal areas where you need to change your study habits, and a rejection from a job can lead you to discover skills you need to develop, or new career paths that might suit you better. This mindset encourages you to ask yourself, "What can I learn from this experience?" rather than "Why did this happen to me?"

Be Positive

Building resilience in these challenges is 'about bouncing forward not back. Reframing your failures involves looking beyond the immediate disappointment and focusing on using the experience to better yourself. Techniques like cognitive restructuring can be helpful here. This involves consciously replacing self-critical thoughts or irrational beliefs about failure with more positive and realistic ones. For example, instead of thinking, "I always mess things up," you might tell yourself, "I faced a tough situation and didn't get the outcome I wanted, but I can use this experience to improve and grow."

Process Your Emotions

Processing the emotions that come with rejection and failure is equally essential. It's okay to feel upset, frustrated, or disappointed. These are natural reactions. However, it's important not to dwell on these emotions for too long. Techniques like expressive writing can be a powerful tool for emotional processing. Writing about your feelings and the experience of rejection can help you clarify your thoughts, reduce stress, and gain new perspectives. Alternatively, talking things out with someone you trust—whether a friend, family member, or counselor—can provide support, reduce feelings of isolation, and help you navigate your emotions more effectively.

Take Action

When it comes to moving forward after a setback, action is critical. Start by setting new, achievable goals that motivate you and give you a sense of direction. These goals don't have to be monumental. They can be as simple as improving a specific skill or exploring a new hobby. What's important is that these goals are meaningful to *you* and reflect what you've learned from your experiences of failure and rejection. Also, consider exploring alternative pathways that might not have occurred to you before. Sometimes, rejection can open unexpected doors, leading to opportunities that align even more closely with your interests and talents.

Maintaining confidence in your abilities and worth is crucial during this phase. Your value doesn't diminish because of setbacks or the opinions of others. Continue to invest in yourself through education, personal development, or simply taking care of your mental and physical health. Over time, these investments build a solid foundation of self-esteem and resilience, making you better equipped to handle future challenges.

As you navigate setbacks and rejections, remember that each experience contributes to your growth and development, no matter how tough. By learning from these situations, processing your emotions healthily, and taking proactive steps forward, you transform potential stumbling blocks into steppingstones, paving your path to success and fulfillment.

Coping with failure and rejection is integral to your growth journey. These experiences, while challenging, teach resilience, foster emotional intelligence, and encourage a proactive approach to life's inevitable ups and downs.

Transitioning from high school to college or taking on new roles in life can feel like a giant leap into the unknown, filled with excitement and challenges. This chapter has equipped you with strategies to anticipate and manage these transitions. By preparing emotionally, developing independence, balancing personal goals with external expectations, embracing new responsibilities, and learning to cope with setbacks, you can navigate these changes with confidence. Each transition is an opportunity for growth, and with the right tools and mindset, you can thrive in your new environment and continue to build a fulfilling and successful life.

As you move forward, remember that every big change begins with a single step, and you have the tools to make that step a successful one. As we transition to the next chapter, we'll explore how maintaining emotional well-being through mindfulness can further enhance your ability to manage life's challenges, ensuring you recover from setbacks and thrive.

In this chapter, we've explored the complex journey of transitioning from high school to college and embracing new roles and responsibilities. We've learned about the importance of emotional preparation, developing independence, and managing expectations—both our own and those of others. We've discussed strategies for prioritizing tasks, setting boundaries, and effectively navigating role conflicts. Additionally, we've explored how to cope with failure and rejection, viewing these experiences as opportunities for growth and learning.

Remember, transitions are challenging but also filled with opportunities for personal development. By applying these strategies—from effective communication and time management to resilience-building and self-reflection—you can navigate these changes more confidently. As you move forward, embrace each new experience as a chance to learn, grow, and become more self-aware, setting the foundation for success in your evolving roles and responsibilities.

Chapter 14
Special Topics in Teen Coping

I magine standing before a colossal canvas, paintbrush in hand, with every shade of paint at your disposal. Now, picture that every color represents a different aspect of who you are—your passions, fears, dreams, and deepest values. Painting this canvas can be likened to the journey of self-discovery. It's about exploring and affirming your identity, a vibrant spectrum of self that includes your sexuality, gender, cultural heritage, and personal values. This chapter delves into how embracing every hue of your identity enriches your life and strengthens your emotional health.

14.1 Navigating Identity and Self-Discovery

The exploration of personal identity is essential for emotional well-being. It involves delving into the elements that make you unique, including your sexuality, gender identity, cultural roots, and the values you hold dear. Understanding and affirming your identity is more than just knowing these aspects. It's about embracing and expressing them in a way that feels true to you. This self-awareness is crucial because it influences how you perceive yourself and, in turn, how you interact with the world. It's the lens through which you view your experiences and make decisions, from the friends you choose to the ambitions you pursue.

This process isn't just about looking inward. It's also about how different parts of your identity connect with each other and the world around you. Understanding your cultural heritage can give you a sense of community, while exploring your gender identity can help you feel more authentic. Each piece of your identity builds a complete picture of who you are, leading to greater confidence and a more fulfilled life.

Challenges in Self-Discovery

The path to self-discovery has its obstacles. Teens often face expectations that may seem at odds with their emerging sense of self. These expectations come from various sources like media, peers, and even family, each potentially pulling you in different directions. For example, societal norms often dictate certain behaviors or roles based on gender, which can be confusing if your own identity doesn't align with these expectations. Similarly, peer pressure can sway you to suppress unique aspects of yourself in favor of fitting in.

Navigating these pressures requires strategies that allow you to remain true to yourself. One practical approach is setting clear personal boundaries that help manage the influence of external opinions. Developing critical thinking skills that allow you to question and challenge societal norms is also helpful. Engaging in open dialogues with trusted individuals can provide support and validation as you explore different facets of your identity.

Role of Experiences in Shaping Identity

Your experiences play a pivotal role in shaping your identity. Diverse experiences such as traveling, pursuing education, and building friendships broaden your perspectives and help you understand and define your own identity in relation to the world. For instance, traveling can expose you to new cultures, influencing your cultural identity and values. Educational experiences can challenge your viewpoints, encourage personal growth, and refine your interests. Friendships, particularly supportive and affirming, can enable you to express your true self and explore aspects of your identity in a safe environment.

Support Systems for Identity Exploration

Finding supportive communities and resources is crucial in your journey of self-discovery. These support systems provide a safe space for exploring your identity without judgment. Cultural organizations can connect you with your heritage, offering a deeper understanding of your background and its impact on your identity. Counseling services can provide guidance and support as you navigate the complexities of self-discovery, helping you to deal with any emotional challenges that arise along the way. For LGBTQ+ youth, centers and online communities can offer crucial support and validation from others with similar experiences.

Identity Exploration Chart

To aid in your exploration of identity, consider creating an Identity Exploration Chart. This tool can help you map out the different aspects of your identity, including your interests, values, cultural background, and how they intersect. Use colors, symbols, or words to represent each aspect and connect them to see how they influence one another. This chart is a reflective tool and a celebration of the complexity and richness of who you are.

Navigating the intricacies of identity and self-discovery is like continuously adding to and refining a painting. Each stroke and color adds depth and authenticity, empowering you to live freely and true to yourself.

14.2 Dealing with Grief and Loss

Imagine you're sitting in your room, surrounded by memories that suddenly feel distant, like echoes of laughter that have faded into silence. Grief is the emotional response to loss, and it's not just about the death of a loved one. It can encompass the heartache from a breakup, the loneliness of moving away from friends, or the unsettling quiet that follows the end of a significant chapter in your life, such as graduating from high school. Understanding grief in its various forms is crucial because it helps validate that your feelings are normal, regardless of the type of loss you're experiencing.

Grief is often depicted as a linear journey with distinct stages. Still, it's more like being in the ocean, where waves of different emotions wash over you, sometimes calm and sometimes overwhelming. The well-known phases of grief—denial, anger, bargaining, depression, and acceptance—are not steps on a ladder but rather responses that can come in any order, sometimes circling back multiple times.

Denial might come as disbelief ("This can't be happening"), followed perhaps by anger ("Why is this happening?"), and then bargaining ("Maybe if I had done something differently"). Depression might follow as the weight of the loss truly sinks in, eventually leading to acceptance—not that the loss is okay, but that it is a reality with which you must live. Recognizing these phases can help you understand that what you're feeling is a normal part of grieving and that it's okay not to be okay for a while.

Creative Expression In Grief

In navigating through grief, finding healthy coping mechanisms is critical. One powerful way is through creative expression—art, writing, or music—which provides an outlet for the emotions that are often too complex to articulate.

Creating something amid your pain can be incredibly thera-peutic. It's like each brush stroke on a canvas, or each word in a diary, acts as a minor release of the emotional pressure that builds up inside. Similarly, music can resonate with your soul, echoing your innermost feelings and help you process your emotions. Engaging in these activities doesn't just help pass the time but facilitates healing.

Support

Connecting with others who have experienced similar losses can also provide comfort and understanding. Whether it's a support group, an online community, or just a friend, who has been through something similar, sharing your feelings with someone who truly understands can be incredibly vali-dating. It reminds you that you're not alone in your journey through grief. Moreover, for those who find their emotions too overwhelming or if grief is significantly impacting their ability to function, seeking professional help from a coun-selor or therapist is a vital step. These professionals can offer strategies tailored to your situation, helping you navigate your grief more effectively.

Maintaining a Connection

For those mourning the death of a loved one, maintaining a connection with the deceased can be an essential part of the healing process. Creating a memory box filled with items that remind you of your loved one, or participating in remembrance activities, can keep your memory alive. This might include lighting a candle on significant dates, visiting places unique to you both, or continuing a tradition they started.

Over time, these actions can transform your relationship with the deceased from presence to memory, allowing you to keep their legacy alive in a personal and meaningful way. By honoring these memories, you're acknowledging that, although the person is gone, their impact on your life remains. This can be a comforting and powerful way to integrate your loss into your life as you move forward.

14.3 Overcoming Fear of Missing Out (FOMO)

Have you ever scrolled through your social media feeds and felt like everyone else's life is packed with exciting events, leaving you feeling like you're just on the sidelines? That creeping sense of being left out is known as Fear of Missing Out or FOMO. It's the anxious feeling that others might be having rewarding experiences without you, and the highlights reel often intensifies what we see on social media platforms. This phenomenon isn't just about a minor case of envy. It's a state that can lead to significant anxiety, affecting your mood, and how you view your own life.

The Risks

FOMO can make you feel like you're not doing enough, or that your life isn't as interesting as others. It can spiral into a loop, where you're constantly seeking something better, or perpetually glued to your devices to check what everyone else is doing. This constant comparison can chip away at your self-esteem and increase feelings of inadequacy. Over time, if left unchecked, it can contribute to more severe issues like anxiety and depression because the life you're comparing to your own isn't even the whole story—it's a curated, often embellished version of reality.

Proactive Steps

To combat FOMO, taking proactive steps toward grounding yourself in your own experiences is vital. One effective strategy is setting limits on how much time you spend on social media. This doesn't mean you have to quit cold turkey but consider designated times during the day when you consciously choose to log off and engage with the natural world instead.

Another approach is to focus on being present. Whether during a meal with family or a hangout with friends, fully immerse yourself in the experience instead of thinking about what else you could do. This mindfulness can enrich your interactions and make your life feel more fulfilling.

Gratitude

Cultivating gratitude is another powerful antidote to FOMO. Take time each day to reflect on things for which you're thankful. This could be as simple as a good book, a pet's companionship, or a nice meal. Gratitude shifts your focus from what you think you lack to the abundance already in your life. Additionally, engaging in activities that align with your interests and values can help mitigate feelings of missing out. When you spend time doing things that genuinely resonate with you, the need to compare or feel left out tends to diminish.

Real Connections in the Real World

Building authentic connections in the real world also plays a crucial role in overcoming FOMO. While it's easy to feel connected to hundreds or even thousands of online friends, more is needed than the depth of face-to-face interactions. Invest time in nurturing relationships that make you feel supported and valued. Real-world interactions can be incredibly grounding and remind you that connection is about quality, not quantity. Engage in community activities, join clubs that interest you, or spend more time with family and friends. These interactions provide a sense of belonging and community that no online platform can replicate.

By actively disconnecting from online portrayals and reconnecting with your immediate world, you can dismantle FOMO's hold on your life. This shift not only enhances your mental health but also deepens your appreciation for your unique path, fostering a life of genuine satisfaction and fewer regrets about what could have been.

14.4 Handling Sudden Fame or Attention

Imagine one day you wake up, and your life has completely flipped—suddenly, everyone knows your name, and your face is all over social media and news outlets. While it might sound like a dream, sudden fame can feel more like a whirlwind, pulling you into a vortex of new demands and expectations. The emotional and psychological challenges accompanying sudden fame, such as privacy invasion, increased scrutiny, and the pressure to maintain a public image, can be overwhelming. Suddenly, your every move is watched, and every word you say can be scrutinized, leading to a sense of loss of privacy that many find daunting.

Boundaries (Again)

Maintaining a sense of normality becomes a critical challenge. Establishing boundaries that help delineate your public and private lives is essential. This could mean setting clear limits with the media, deciding what parts of your life you want to share, and what should remain private. Prioritizing close relationships is also crucial. These people knew you before your rise to fame and can help keep you grounded. They remind you of your roots and can provide stability amidst the chaos of fame. Moreover, sticking to routine activities you've always enjoyed—morning runs, weekly coffee at your favorite cafe, or movie nights with friends—can help maintain a sense of continuity in your life.

Public Perception

Managing public perception is another significant aspect of dealing with fame. How you interact with the public and handle criticism can significantly impact your image. Constructive handling of criticism is essential. Listen' to feedback without letting it define you. Not all critiques are worth your attention, and learning to differentiate constructive feedback from mere trolling is critical. Additionally, how you use your platforms matters immensely. Being responsible about what you post, understanding your influence, and using your platform to advocate for causes you care about can shape public perception positively and give you a sense of purpose.

Professional Guidance

Seeking professional guidance is often necessary to navigate the complexities of sudden fame. Public relations managers can help manage your image and interactions with the media, ensuring your public persona aligns with your values. Moreover, talking to a mental health counselor can be invaluable in dealing with the stress and emotional upheaval that fame can bring. These professionals can provide strategies to cope with stress, handle public scrutiny, and maintain mental health.

Navigating sudden fame is like learning to sail in stormy waters—challenging but not impossible with the right strategies and support. By setting boundaries, maintaining normalcy, managing public interactions carefully, and seeking professional advice, you can successfully navigate these waters, ensuring that your new-found fame does not overwhelm your personal life or sense of self.

This chapter has explored various aspects of teen coping, focusing on identity and self-discovery, navigating grief and loss, overcoming the fear of missing out (FOMO), and handling sudden fame or attention. By understanding and embracing your unique identity, finding healthy ways to cope with grief, grounding yourself in your own experiences, and setting boundaries in the face of fame, you can build resilience and emotional strength. These strategies not only help you navigate the challenges of adolescence but also empower you to live a more balanced and fulfilling life.

Chapter 15
Empowering Actions for Everyday Life

Imagine waking up to a day where every step you take is deliberate and geared toward stabilizing your emotional world. From the moment you open your eyes to the moment you lay your head down to sleep, each action you perform can fortify your mental peace and create a reservoir of emotional energy that fuels you through ups and downs. This isn't just a fantasy—it's achievable with the proper daily habits. In this chapter, we'll explore how routines, physical activity, reflection, and sleep can be woven into the fabric of your everyday life to enhance your emotional stability and overall well-being.

15.1 Daily Habits for Emotional Stability

The tone of your entire day can often be set in the first hour after you wake up. Establishing a morning routine is like laying down the first card in a house of cards with precision —it sets the foundation for building a stable structure. Start your day with practices that ground you and fill you with positivity.

Consider beginning with a few minutes of meditation to clear your mind and center your thoughts. Meditation can be as simple as sitting quietly and focusing on your breath or using guided meditations from a mobile app. Follow this with a healthy breakfast that fuels your body with the nutrients it needs to tackle the day. While you eat, set your intentions for the day. What do you want to achieve? What kind of attitude do you want to maintain? These morning rituals give a structured start to your day and empower you to handle whatever comes your way with a calm, focused mind.

Regular Physical Activity

The link between physical activity and mental health is well-documented and profound. Regular exercise can act as a natural antidepressant, enhancing mood and dissipating stress. Unless that's what you enjoy, it doesn't have to mean hitting the gym or running marathons. Integrating activities like walking, cycling, dancing, or participating in team sports into your daily life can significantly impact your emotional well-being.

These activities release endorphins, often known as 'feel-good' hormones, which can lift your mood and provide a sense of accomplishment. Make it a goal to move your body for at least thirty minutes daily. If that fits your schedule better, you can break this time into shorter segments. Remember, the best kind of exercise for you is the one you enjoy and can consistently incorporate into your life.

Nightly Reflection

Just as you start your day with intention, ending it with reflection can offer insights into your emotional patterns and help you process the day's events. Spend a few minutes each night journaling or meditating. Reflect on what went well, and what challenges you encountered. What emotions did you feel the strongest? How did you respond to stressful situations? This practice is not about critiquing your day but understanding and acknowledging your experiences. It helps you recognize your strengths, and areas where you want to grow. This nightly routine can also serve as a wind-down process, signaling to your brain that it's time to slow down and prepare for rest.

Consistent Sleep Schedule

Sleep is as crucial to your mental health as food and water are to your physical health. A consistent sleep schedule helps regulate your body's internal clock and improves the quality of your sleep. Aim for seven to nine hours of sleep per night. Try to go to bed and wake up at the same time every day, even on weekends. Create a bedtime routine that promotes relaxation, such as reading a book, listening to soothing music, or taking a warm bath. Avoid screens at least an hour before bed, as the blue light emitted can interfere with melatonin production, the hormone responsible for regulating sleep.

By integrating these practices into your daily life, you create a framework that supports your emotional well-being. Such routines stabilize your mood and empower you to manage life's stresses with resilience and grace. The goal is not to perfect these practices but to make them a consistent part of your life, adapting them as your needs and circumstances change.

15.2 Setting and Achieving Personal Emotional Goals

When you think about where you want to be regarding your emotional health, what comes to mind? It could be feeling less overwhelmed by school stress or being able to bounce back quicker from disappointments. Setting personal emotional goals isn't just about reducing negative feelings. It's about enhancing your overall quality of life, making each day more vibrant and fulfilling. Let's break down how you can define clear and achievable emotional goals, plan actionable steps toward these goals, monitor your progress, and adjust your strategies as needed.

Define Your Emotional Goals

Defining your personal emotional goals is the first step toward a more balanced and satisfying emotional life. Start by identifying areas in your emotional landscape that feel rocky. For instance, do you find yourself frequently overwhelmed by stress? Are there moments when you wish you had handled a situation more calmly? These reflections can guide you to specific, achievable goals, such as improving stress management, or enhancing your ability to remain calm under pressure. It's essential to frame your goals positively. Instead of setting a goal like "stop feeling anxious," aim for "develop strategies to manage anxiety during exams." This positive framing sets a clear direction and makes the journey toward achieving these goals more motivating and empowering.

Plan Steps

Planning steps to achieve your goals involves breaking down each goal into manageable, actionable steps. Begin by setting short-term objectives that will lead you toward your larger goal. For example, if your goal is to manage stress better, a short-term objective might be practicing mindfulness for five minutes daily. Next, identify potential obstacles you might encounter, such as a busy schedule that could make it hard to find time for mindfulness. Planning for these challenges by determining the resources needed, such as using a meditation app that guides you through quick, practical sessions, will prepare you to overcome them. Consistency is the key. Small daily efforts can lead to significant emotional growth over time.

Track Progress

Monitoring progress is essential to understand how well you are doing in achieving your emotional goals. This could involve regular check-ins with yourself through journaling or using apps that track mood and emotional health. Documenting your feelings daily can help you see patterns contributing to, or detracting from, your emotional well-being—for instance, your stress levels are lower on days when you meditate or engage in physical activity. These insights are valuable as they guide you on what's working and what isn't, helping you to fine-tune your approach continuously.

Adjust as Needed

Adjusting goals as needed is an integral part of the process. As you progress, your initial goals may evolve or change completely, and that's okay. Flexibility is crucial. If a particular technique isn't working for you, be willing to try something new. Similarly, if you achieve a goal, set a new one that helps you continue to grow. This ongoing adjustment keeps your approach fresh and ensures your emotional health strategies align with your changing life circumstances. Most importantly, approach these adjustments with self-compassion. Recognize that growth often involves learning from what doesn't work as much as what does.

By setting clear emotional goals, planning actionable steps, monitoring your progress, and being flexible, you actively empower yourself to shape your emotional landscape. This proactive stance on emotional well-being can transform challenges into steppingstones toward greater resilience and happiness. As you continue to engage in this process, remember that each step forward, no matter how small, is a crucial part of your journey toward a more emotionally fulfilling life.

15.3 Using Technology for Mental Health: Apps and Tools

In this digital era, where screens often dominate our daily interactions, it's refreshing to know that technology can also be a powerful ally in managing mental health. Various apps designed to support mental well-being have become invaluable tools for many. These include meditation apps that guide you through calming exercises, mood trackers that help you monitor your emotional trends, and cognitive-behavioral therapy (CBT) apps that offer strategies to manage anxiety and stress. Each app is crafted to provide unique support, whether helping you find peace in a hectic day or providing insights into patterns in your mood.

Mental Health Apps

When considering which mental health apps to integrate into your life, choosing those that align with your specific needs and preferences is crucial. Start by identifying what you want to improve or manage more effectively—stress, sleep, anxiety, or mood swings. Once you have a clear idea, explore highly rated apps for these purposes. Reading user reviews and checking the privacy policies of these apps is essential, as you want to ensure that your data is protected and the app's functionalities genuinely benefit your mental health. Here are some highly recommended apps:

Headspace: Offers guided meditation sessions and mindfulness techniques.

https://www.headspace.com

Calm: Provides guided meditations, sleep stories, and relaxation techniques.

https://www.calm.com

Moodfit: Helps track mood and provides tools for managing anxiety and depression.

https://www.getmoodfit.com

Sanvello: Combines CBT, mindfulness, and mood tracking for managing anxiety and depression.

https://www.sanvello.com

Youper: An AI-powered assistant that offers emotional health support and tracking.

https://www.youper.ai

Happify: Uses science-based activities and games to reduce stress and build resilience.

https://www.happify.com

Woebot: An AI chatbot that provides CBT-based techniques for managing mental health.

https://woebothealth.com

Selecting the right app can provide you with the tools and support needed to enhance your mental well-being effectively.

Integrating these apps into your daily routine can be a game-changer. For instance, start your morning with a guided meditation from Headspace to set a calm tone for the day. Use a mood-tracking app to note emotional fluctuations throughout the day, which can help you identify triggers and patterns. Before bed, turning to a sleep app that plays soothing sounds could help you wind down and prepare for a restful night. The key is consistency; these apps are most effective when used regularly. Think of them as part of your mental health toolkit, always within reach and ready to assist when you need support.

Be Aware of Limitations

While these apps offer significant benefits, they are not a panacea. Awareness of the limitations of using apps for mental health is essential. They should not replace professional help if you are dealing with severe mental health issues. Apps can be fantastic for providing support and daily tools, but they work best when used with traditional therapy and medical advice when necessary.

Remember, these tools are part of a broader approach to mental wellness that includes lifestyle changes, treatment, and, sometimes, medication. Being proactive about your mental health involves utilizing technology as one of many resources that help you navigate the complexities of your emotional landscape more quickly and confidently.

15.4 Advocating for Mental Health in Your Community

Advocating for mental health isn't just about supporting those who are struggling. It's about changing how society views and handles mental health issues. It means raising awareness, reducing stigma, and fostering a community that supports mental wellness openly and actively. When you advocate for mental health, you're helping others by promoting understanding and acceptance, empowering yourself, and contributing to a more compassionate society.

Be an Advocate

Let's start with what it means to be an advocate. In the context of mental health, advocacy can involve anything from educating peers about mental health issues to supporting more significant initiatives that aim to improve mental health services. It's about speaking up and taking action through writing, speaking, or simply being an informed and supportive friend or family member. Advocacy is powerful because it not only helps break down the stigma associated with mental health challenges but also builds a more robust support network for everyone.

How to Start

Starting small is an excellent way for you to begin your advocacy journey. Consider leveraging blogs or social media platforms to share your experiences or essential information about mental health. Social media can be a double-edged sword, but it's a powerful tool for spreading messages quickly and widely.

You could create posts that share how to recognize signs of mental health issues, offer supportive responses, or debunk common myths about mental health. Participating in, or starting, initiatives in your school, such as workshops or awareness campaigns, can also significantly impact you. These efforts help create an environment where students feel more comfortable discussing mental health and seeking help when needed.

Support Groups

Another effective way to advocate is by joining or forming support groups. These groups provide a safe space for individuals to share their experiences, offer support, and feel less alone. If your school doesn't already have a mental health club or support group, consider starting one. You can collaborate with school counselors or teachers to set it up and ensure it provides meaningful support. These groups can also organize events, bring in speakers, or provide resources that educate and inform your community about mental health.

The Next Level

Engaging in more significant initiatives can be incredibly

fulfilling for those ready to take their advocacy to the next level. This might include participating in national mental health awareness campaigns or collaborating with local mental health organizations. These activities often provide opportunities to work on larger projects, such as policy advocacy or community-wide events, which can lead to significant changes in public perceptions and policy. Your involvement could include fundraising for mental health causes or volunteering at local mental health clinics or hotlines. By engaging with these initiatives, you contribute to broad societal change and gain a deeper understanding of the complexities of mental health challenges and the systems that address them.

Advocating for mental health is about making a difference in your community, big or small. It's about using your voice and actions to help change the narrative around mental health, making it okay to talk about, seek help for, and support each other through mental health challenges. As a teen, your advocacy can inspire others, including adults, to take action and show that mental health is a vital part of overall well-being that deserves attention and respect. By stepping up as an advocate, you contribute to a culture of care and understanding that can support everyone's mental health journey.

15.5 Keeping an Emotional Journal: Why and How

Imagine having a personal space to unload thoughts, navigate your emotions, and reflect on your daily experiences without judgment. Keeping an emotional journal can be that haven. It's like having a dialogue with your deepest self, where you can express frustrations, celebrate successes, and ponder life's various shades. Writing down your feelings isn't just about recording events'. It can be a therapeutic process that enhances self-awareness, reduces stress, and improves your ability to process emotions.

Benefits

The benefits of keeping an emotional journal are profound. Firstly, it serves as a mirror reflecting your internal world, helping you better understand your emotional responses and triggers. This heightened self-awareness can lead to better control over your reactions and help you manage your emotional health proactively. Furthermore, journaling has been found to significantly reduce stress, as it allows you to clarify your thoughts and feelings and grapple with them tangibly. Writing can also be immensely cathartic, releasing bottled-up emotions essential for maintaining mental health.

How to Start

Getting started with journaling can be as simple as picking a notebook that resonates with you and deciding when you feel most inclined to write. The key is consistency. Choose an inviting journal—maybe it has a cover that calms or inspires you. As for when to write, some find that journaling in the morning helps them set the tone for the day ahead, while others prefer the evening as it allows them to reflect on the day's events. Finding a quiet, comfortable space, where you won't be disturbed, is crucial. This space should feel safe and private, a personal retreat where you can open up without fear of interruption or oversight.

Prompting

Journal prompts can be incredibly helpful when staring at a blank page, unsure of what to write. They can guide your thoughts and encourage a deeper exploration of your emotions. Here are some prompts to get you started:

- What moment today brought me the most joy, and why?
- What situation stressed me out today, and how did I handle it?
- Am I holding onto something I need to let go of? What steps can I take to release it?
- What is one thing I accomplished today of which I am proud?
- Who or what made me feel appreciated today, and how did it affect my mood?
- What are three things I am grateful for today?
- How did I take care of myself today?
- What is one thing I learned about myself today?

These prompts aren't just questions but gateways to deeper introspection, helping you uncover patterns in your emotional responses and identify areas of your life that may need more attention or adjustment.

Regular journaling can transform the way you understand and interact with your emotions. It's not just about venting frustrations; it's about discovering who you are beneath the day-to-day noise. As you continue to journal, you likely notice subtle shifts in your approach to challenges and changes in how you perceive your emotional reactions. This ongoing practice fosters a greater understanding of yourself and equips you with the tools to navigate the complexities of emotions with more ease and confidence. Each entry builds on the last, forming a comprehensive narrative of your emotional evolution—a narrative that is uniquely yours.

15.6 Preparing for Adulthood: Emotional Skills for Life

Navigating the shift from teenage years to adulthood is like upgrading to a new software version. It's exciting but comes with many updates and debugging. As you stand on the threshold of adulthood, your life's landscape extends far beyond the high school corridors into realms where independence, responsibilities, and broader social interactions play crucial roles. The emotional skills you cultivate now, such as resilience, empathy, self-regulation, and conflict resolution, are the tools that will help you navigate this new terrain successfully.

Resilience

Resilience, the ability to bounce back from setbacks, is more than just recovering from a failed test or a breakup; it's about handling job rejections, financial stress, or personal loss in the future. Developing resilience involves embracing challenges as opportunities for growth and learning from each experience. Empathy, the ability to understand and share the feelings of another, is crucial as you build deeper relationships, both professionally and personally. It allows you to see beyond your perspective and connect with people genuinely, fostering meaningful interactions and support systems.

Self-Regulation

Self-regulation refers to managing your thoughts, emotions, and behaviors constructively. As adult life introduces higher stakes and pressures, self-regulation helps you control impulses, manage stress, and stay aligned with your long-term goals.

Conflict Resolution

Conflict resolution is another vital skill essential for navigating disagreements in both personal and professional settings. Effective conflict resolution involves clear communication, understanding multiple perspectives, finding mutually beneficial solutions, and ensuring that relationships are maintained rather than damaged by disputes.

Big Changes

Significant emotional challenges mark the transition from teen to adult life. Increased responsibilities like managing finances or living alone require new levels of independence and self-sufficiency. The support networks you relied on may change as friends move away from college or jobs and as family dynamics shift. This transition period is critical to actively apply your emotional skills, ensuring you adapt and thrive in your new adult roles.

Consider common life scenarios you might face soon: Starting a new job, managing your finances, or moving out independently. Each scenario requires specific emotional strategies. For instance, starting a new job might bring anxiety and the need for assertiveness. Practicing self-regulation by setting personal boundaries and managing stress through techniques like mindfulness can make the transition smoother. When managing finances, resilience plays a crucial role in handling the stress of budgeting and the potential setbacks of unexpected expenses. Setting up a financial plan and monitoring your spending can be practical applications of this skill.

Living alone for the first time can be challenging but also an exciting opportunity to demonstrate independence. Ensuring you maintain a support network, even if it's through digital means, can help manage feelings of loneliness or isolation. Regular check-ins with family or friends, joining local or online communities, and engaging in social activities can keep you connected. During this significant change, developing routines that incorporate self-care practices can also stabilize your emotional health.

Maintaining emotional health into adulthood is an ongoing process that requires attention and care. Continual self-care, lifelong learning, and seeking professional help when needed are all part of nurturing your emotional well-being.

Self-care practices like regular physical activity, balanced nutrition, and adequate sleep are just as important in adulthood as during your teenage years. Lifelong learning, such as pursuing further education, attending workshops, or reading extensively, keeps your mind engaged and responsive. It also helps you adapt to changes in your personal life and career. There might be times when the challenges of adult life feel overwhelming, and it's important to recognize when professional help is needed. Seeking therapy or counseling during such times is not a sign of weakness but a proactive step toward maintaining your mental health.

Navigating adulthood is an exciting journey that brings its own set of challenges and rewards. By developing and applying critical emotional skills, you equip yourself to handle the complexities of adult life with confidence and resilience. These skills enhance your ability to cope with immediate challenges and lay the groundwork for sustained emotional well-being throughout your life.

15.7 The Role of Emotional Intelligence in Career Success

Navigating the intricate web of professional life demands more than technical skills or academic knowledge. It requires robust emotional intelligence (EI) skills that can significantly influence your career trajectory and leadership capabilities. Imagine stepping into a workplace where your work output and ability to understand, empathize, and effectively interact with others shape your professional success. This is where emotional intelligence comes into play, integrating skills such as empathy, self-regulation, and adept interpersonal communication to create a work environment that thrives on mutual respect and understanding.

A Bridge

Emotional intelligence in the workplace acts as a bridge between meeting personal goals and achieving professional efficiency. For instance, empathy allows you to understand your colleagues' perspectives and challenges, fostering a supportive team environment. Self-regulation helps you manage your emotions, even in high-stress situations, ensuring you can make thoughtful decisions and maintain a professional demeanor. Interpersonal communication skills are crucial for clear and compelling exchanges of ideas, feedback, and instructions, all of which are essential for successful collaboration. These EI skills are desirable; they often distinguish highly respected leaders from the rest.

Development

Developing these emotional intelligence skills professionally involves continuous practice and conscious effort. Start by seeking feedback from peers and mentors about your interaction styles and emotional responses. Use this feedback to identify areas for improvement, such as working on your patience, or becoming more receptive to constructive criticism.

Engage in role-playing exercises that can help you practice and enhance your communication and conflict-resolution skills. Workshops and training sessions on EI development can also provide valuable tools and insights. Another effective strategy is to take on diverse team projects that expose you to various interpersonal dynamics and challenges, giving you practical experience in adapting and applying your emotional intelligence in real-world settings.

Aligned Values

Aligning personal values with professional goals is another dimension of emotional intelligence that can lead to a more fulfilling career. This alignment ensures that your career path meets your financial or professional aspirations and resonates with your personal beliefs and values, leading to greater job satisfaction and reduced workplace stress. Reflect on what values are most important to you, such as integrity, creativity, or community, and seek out roles or companies that echo these values. This unity can motivate you to invest more deeply in your work and contribute to a positive workplace culture.

Important in Every Career

The importance of emotional intelligence transcends industries and job roles. For example, in healthcare, professionals with high EI can better empathize with patients, leading to improved patient care and satisfaction. In fields like marketing or customer service, understanding and anticipating client emotions can enhance service delivery and client retention. In leadership roles across all sectors, emotional intelligence is crucial for managing teams effectively, resolving conflicts, and steering complex projects to success. These examples underscore how emotional intelligence is a critical, universal asset that plays a significant role in a wide range of professional scenarios, enhancing not just individual careers but also the overall health of organizations.

By focusing on nurturing your emotional intelligence, you equip yourself with the tools to succeed in your chosen career and to lead with compassion, understanding, and efficiency. As you progress in your professional journey, these skills will continue to serve as your foundation, enabling you to navigate the complexities of the workplace with confidence and poise.

15.8 Continuous Learning and Emotional Growth

Learning is a lifelong journey—yes, that's right, even after you've tossed your graduation cap and said goodbye to school. But here's the twist: Continuous learning isn't just about accumulating knowledge but about expanding your emotional intelligence and adaptability, which are vital to maintaining your emotional well-being.

Think of it as updating the apps on your phone. You're essentially upgrading your mind and emotional toolkit to navigate life's complexities better. Embracing an attitude of curiosity and openness to new experiences can significantly enhance your ability to handle life's inevitable ups and downs with more grace and resilience.

The world is your classroom, with countless resources available to facilitate your continuous emotional education. Books can be a window into the minds and experiences of others, offering new perspectives and insights that challenge your perceptions and beliefs. Online courses on platforms like Coursera or Khan Academy, and workshops or seminars focused on personal development and emotional intelligence, provide structured learning opportunities that can deepen your understanding of yourself and the world around you. These resources often cover a variety of topics, from stress management and mindfulness to more complex subjects like cognitive behavioral therapy techniques. Engaging with these materials can open up new avenues for personal growth and emotional management that you might not have considered before.

Integration

Integrating this new knowledge into your daily life is where the real magic happens. It's not enough to consume information. You must apply it to see fundamental changes. Start by setting small, achievable goals for implementing new strategies. For example, if you learn a new technique for managing stress, practice it at the first sign of tension. Keep a log of what you know and how you apply it, noting what works and what doesn't. This practice can help you adapt the techniques to suit your needs and lifestyle better. Discussing what you've learned with friends or mentors can reinforce your new knowledge and inspire others to engage in their learning journeys.

Reflective Practice

Reflective practice is a powerful tool for sustained emotional growth. It involves regularly taking stock of your experiences and the emotions they evoke. Consider setting aside time each week to reflect on what you've learned and how you've grown. This could be through meditation, journaling, or simply quiet contemplation. Use questions like, "What new things did I learn about myself this week?" or "How have I handled emotional challenges differently?" These reflections can provide profound insights into your growth and help you navigate your emotional landscape with increasing adeptness.

Embracing lifelong learning as a strategy for emotional well-being encourages a dynamic approach to personal development. It ensures you are always equipped with the latest tools and information to manage your emotional health, adapt to changes, and lead a fulfilling life. By continually seeking to learn and grow, you enhance your own life and enrich the lives of those around you. This chapter invites you to step into a world where learning is an ongoing adventure—one that nurtures your mind, fortifies your heart, and elevates your spirit.

Conclusion

As we reach this journey's final pages, let's reflect on the path we've traversed together. From the outset, we embarked on a comprehensive exploration of our emotional terrains, learning to decode and navigate the complexities of our feelings. We've delved into advanced coping strategies and prepared ourselves for the inevitable challenges.

Throughout this book, we've underscored the critical components of effective teen coping—self-awareness, emotional management, resilience, and cultivating supportive relationships. Each chapter aims to arm you with the knowledge and tools necessary for understanding and managing your emotions, fostering an environment where you can thrive amidst life's ups and downs.

One of the core messages we've revisited time and again is the empowerment that comes from mastering self-regulation tools. These tools are more than just techniques. They are your allies in building a life where you can face challenges with confidence and poise. By integrating therapeutic approaches like Cognitive Behavioral Therapy (CBT) and Dialectical Behavioral Therapy (DBT), we've offered a unique and rich toolkit that addresses a spectrum of emotional needs.

The practical exercises and real-life applicability are not merely academic but meant to be lived, tested, and integrated into your daily routines. Whether through mindfulness practices, structured problem-solving, or emotional journaling, the strategies we've discussed are designed to bring about real change in how you cope with stress, anxiety, and the myriad emotions that color your world.

This book stands out by blending various therapeutic methods, offering a holistic approach to emotional wellness that respects the complexity of your experiences and individuality. As you continue to grow and evolve, so should your strategies for managing emotions and overcoming obstacles.

You should view emotional development as an ongoing journey that doesn't end with the last page of this book. Keep learning, keep reflecting, and keep adapting the strategies you've learned to meet the needs of your changing life.

As you move forward, remember the importance of supportive adults in your journey. Engage with anyone who can provide guidance and support, such as parents, teachers,

Conclusion

or mentors. Their experiences and insights can be invaluable as you navigate the challenges of growing up.

I am hopeful and confident in your ability to manage your emotional landscape. You have the tools, the knowledge, and the resilience to lead a fulfilling and emotionally healthy life. Continue to reach out, explore, and grow. Your potential is boundless, and your capacity for happiness is immense.

Lastly, I invite you to share your experiences and feedback. How has this book helped shape your coping strategies? What challenges have you overcome using the tools discussed? Your stories can inspire and encourage others, fostering a community of growth and shared wisdom.

Thank you for joining me on this meaningful journey. May you move forward with courage, curiosity, and a heart full of hope.

An Invitation

Congratulations on completing The Teen's Coping Toolkit, gaining valuable insights on handling social pressure, managing challenging situations, and boosting self-esteem. Armed with these tools, you're now better equipped to navigate the ups and downs of adolescence.

As you reflect on your journey, consider sharing your experience with others. By leaving a review of this book on Amazon, you can help other teens discover the support and guidance they need to thrive. Your words can inspire and guide others on their path toward personal growth and resilience. Your review has the power to make a difference in the lives of many.

Your contribution is not just valuable; it's essential. Resilience and growth are built on shared knowledge and experiences. Your review supports me as an author and serves as a beacon of hope for those seeking guidance.

Thank you for being an active part of this journey. Your participation is crucial in our mission to empower and uplift teens worldwide.

With heartfelt thanks,

C.M. Krueger

ENJOY YOUR FREE GIFTS

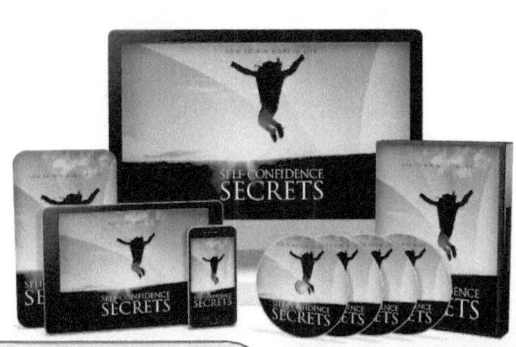

SELF-CONFIDENCE SECRETS COURSE

ANIMAL MANDALA COLORING BOOK

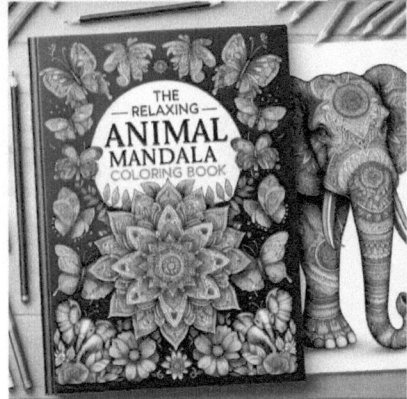

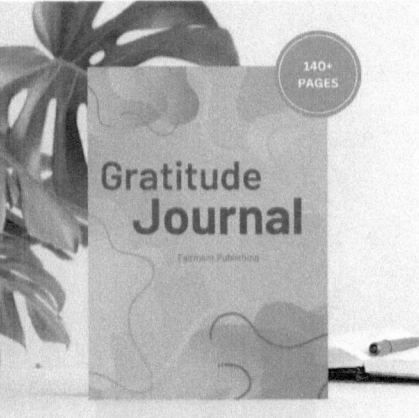

EASY TO USE GRATITUDE JOURNAL

ENJOY!

THANK YOU

Thank You for Your Purchase!

We are truly grateful for your purchase of The Teen's Coping Toolkit! As a token of our appreciation, we are excited to offer you three exclusive thank-you gifts to enhance your journey of personal growth and self-improvement:

1. Self-Confidence Secrets Super Bundle

- Dive into a comprehensive self-confidence training program.
- Includes the Self-Confidence Secrets Guide, Cheat Sheet, Mindmap, and Resources.
- Access an engaging 10-part companion video series to help you grow your self-confidence today!

2. Full-Color Easy to Use Gratitude Journal

- Transform your life with the practice of gratitude.
- Explore 140 pages to build and expand your sense of gratitude.

3. The Relaxing Animal Mandala Coloring Book

- Enjoy 50 spectacularly beautiful animal mandalas designed for your coloring enjoyment.

But wait, there's more! We would love for you to leave a review of The Teen's Coping Toolkit and let us know how it has helped you. Your feedback is invaluable to us and will help others discover the benefits of this fantastic toolkit.

Sign up now by scanning the QR code below or visiting https://fairmontpublishing.com/signup-6563-5324 to receive your thank-you gifts and continue your personal development journey. Thank you for choosing The Teen's Coping Toolkit!

Sources

Teenagers need a wider emotional vocabulary to better express their feelings https://www.abc.net.au/education/teens-need-a-wide-emotional-vocabulary-to-express-their-feelings/14038450

How to Identify Emotional Triggers in 3 Steps https://ridgeviewhospital.net/how-to-identify-emotional-triggers-in-3-steps/

Emotional Development | HHS Office of Population Affairs https://opa.hhs.gov/adolescent-health/adolescent-development-explained/emotional-development#:~:text=Hormones.,decisions%20that%20adults%20find%20app

Journaling for Emotional Wellness https://www.nationwidechildrens.org/family-resources-education/family-resources-library/journaling-for-emotional-wellness

Breathing Techniques for Stress Relief https://www.webmd.com/balance/stress-management/stress-relief-breathing-techniques

My Anxiety Plan (MAP) for Adults | Blog https://www.anxietycanada.com/articles/my-anxiety-plan-map-for-adults/

5 Evidence-Based Anger Management Techniques for Teens https://www.newportacademy.com/resources/empowering-teens/anger-management-techniques/

Activity Scheduling as a Core Component of Effective Care https://www.ncbi.nlm.nih.gov/pmc/articles/PMC3429703/

Mindfulness Exercises (for Teens) | Nemours KidsHealth https://kidshealth.org/en/teens/mindful-exercises.html

Mindfulness for Teens: Benefits and Practice Tips https://psychcentral.com/health/the-benefits-of-mindfulness-meditation-for-teens

Creating a Meditation Space in Your Home https://leftbrainbuddha.com/create-a-meditation-space-in-your-home/

7 mindfulness tips to help students deal with exam stress https://www.acs-schools.com/future-focus-blog/how-can-mindfulness-combat-exam-stress

Cognitive Behavioral Therapy for Teens – A Complete Guide https://clear

Sources

forkacademy.com/blog/cognitive-behavioral-therapy-for-teens-a-complete-guide/

Cognitive Distortions for Teens: Types, Examples, and More https://mental healthcenterkids.com/blogs/articles/cognitive-distortions-for-teens

ABC Model of Cognitive Behavioral Therapy: How it Works https://www.healthline.com/health/abc-model

10 Best Problem-Solving Therapy Worksheets & Activities https://posi tivepsychology.com/problem-solving-therapy/

What Is DBT and How Can It Help Teens? | Newport Academy https://www.newportacademy.com/resources/mental-health/what-is-dbt/#:~:text=DBT%20skills%20for%20teens%20cover,emotion%20regula tion%2C%20and%20interpersonal%20effectiveness.

21 Emotion Regulation Worksheets & Strategies https://positivepsychology.com/emotion-regulation-worksheets-strategies-dbt-skills/

What Are Distress Tolerance Skills? Your Ultimate DBT Toolkit https://positivepsychology.com/distress-tolerance-skills/

Dialectical Behavior Therapy (DBT) for Teens https://www.talkspace.com/blog/dbt-for-teens/

Building Resilience in Children and Teens https://www.newportacademy.com/resources/well-being/resilience-in-teens/

10 Self-esteem Activities for Teens, Worksheets, & Questions https://www.carepatron.com/guides/self-esteem-activities-for-teens

How Using Social Media Affects Teenagers - Child Mind Institute https://childmind.org/article/how-using-social-media-affects-teenagers/#:~:text=Social%20media%20affects%20teenagers'%20-mental,esteem%2C%20anxiety%2C%20and%20depression.

How Perfectionism in Children and Teens Impacts Mental Health https://www.newportacademy.com/resources/empowering-teens/perfection ism-in-children/#:~:text=Educate%20your%20child%20about%20per fectionism.&text=Help%20them%20understand%20its%20true,%2Dcriticism%20with%20self%2Dcompassion.

13 Practical Time Management Skills To Teach Teens https://lifeskillsadvo cate.com/blog/13-practical-time-management-skills-to-teach-teens/

Teens and social media use: What's the impact? https://www.mayoclinic.org/healthy-lifestyle/tween-and-teen-health/in-depth/teens-and-social-media-use/art-20474437

Sources

Empowering Teens: Effective Strategies for Teaching Assertiveness in High School   https://everydayspeech.com/blog-posts/general/empowering-teens-effective-strategies-for-teaching-assertiveness-in-high-school/

CBT vs. DBT | Skyland Trail https://www.skylandtrail.org/4-differences-between-cbt-and-dbt-and-how-to-tell-which-is-right-for-you/#:~:text=CBT%20seeks%20to%20give%20patients,potentially%20destructive%20or%20harmful%20behaviors.